The
Halfway House
Movement
A Search for Sanity

THE CENTURY PSYCHOLOGY SERIES

Richard M. Elliott, Gardner Lindzey
and Kenneth MacCorquodale

Editors

The
Halfway House
Movement
A Search for Sanity

Harold L. Raush
UNIVERSITY OF MICHIGAN

with

Charlotte L. Raush

Appleton
Century
Crofts

New York

DIVISION OF MEREDITH CORPORATION

618-1

Library of Congress Card Number: 68-18037

PRINTED IN THE UNITED STATES OF AMERICA

E72855

To
Joan Doniger
and
Edith Maeda

PREFACE

The history of madness and of the "sane" man's attempt to deal with it is intimately bound with man's conception of himself and his world. Reflected in his view of madness is man's cultural history, his cosmogony, theology and philosophy, his myths and his sciences. Whether the madman is seen as inspired or possessed, whether he is respected as a seer, burned as a witch or sorcerer, enchained as a lunatic, or hospitalized as a patient depends on the time he is born into. And the choice reflects not so much the body of knowledge of these times as it does their spirit.

The story is not yet ended.

Today the mad are called "sick." They suffer a "mental illness" which is "just like any other illness and certainly nothing to be ashamed of." If they are sufficiently disturbing to us, they are put into hospitals, some of which are devoted exclusively to the "treatment" of this "disease." Such hospitals are much like other hospitals—with the wards and beds, with the doctors, nurses, and attendants, and with the complex administrative apparatus of hospitals. In some ways mental hospitals differ from other hospitals, but these differences have not changed our views very much. We still, for example, use the language familiar to hospitals: even when calling for reforms, we are apt to note that "half of all hospital *beds* are occupied by the *mentally ill*."

We have changed our terms for those who seek to guide the mad to pathways of return. No longer are they soothsayers as was David for Saul; no longer are they inquisitors exorcising the devils which infested the souls of the unwary from the Middle Ages to the end of the seventeenth century; no longer are they the puritan churchmen who struggled with the Devil for the souls of witches; no longer are they the tolerant physicians of the early nineteenth century, concerned with the dignity and the moral problems of those whom life had treated too harshly.

The age of science and its medical counterpart ushered in an era of medical treatment for madness. From the industrial revolution came urbanization and growing separation of work from family roles, creating increased difficulties in maintaining the psychologically alienated within the bounds of ordinary society. The mental hospital for the insane—an institution still less than two hundred years old—multiplied and grew in size and in distance from the working community. Furthermore, within the medical cosmogony it seemed reasonable that a syndrome of what are now called symptoms would have a specific etiology and would be subject to a specific course of treatment.

But somehow our system of medical treatment has, like the others, broken down. Notions of brain pathology, toxemias, nutritional deficiencies offered too few solutions to the mystery of madness, and the treatments based on these notions have now gone by the board. Heroic efforts are still being expended toward establishing specific etiologies and discovering specific treatments. But the etiology has given way to *mental* etiology, and the treatment to *mental* treatment.

We are just beginning to explore how daring this leap is. It is an unwilling exploration. We have tried to think of our psychological lives as similar to a collection of bodily organs—as relatively discrete and "treatable." Though faced with contradictions we have been, for the most part, unwilling to open a Pandora's box of new demons. We hold tight to our outmoded but familiar models. We speak of "patients" and "treatment" and "cure." Seeking comfort in familiar medical analogies, in our "treatment" of the mind we "employ" chemotherapy and psychotherapy (individual, group, conjoint and family). We also have in our pharmacopoeia such ancillary "therapies" as rehabilitation therapy, milieu therapy, occupational therapy, recreational therapy, music therapy, dance therapy. And if you recommend a book to someone, that must be bibliotherapy. This proliferation is of course appropriate to our own age of fragmentation, specialization and expertise. Nonetheless the absurdities are being felt.

The notion of a multiplicity of therapies, each competing

for title of "real cure," or all cooperating in the "total treatment"
of an ill-understood disease, is becoming untenable. We are coming
to recognize that, whatever their ultimate cause and etiology, the
problems faced by the deranged concern the trials and vicissitudes
of living in this world with oneself and with others. Those of us
who are not quite mad have the same kinds of problems, and we
too solve them in accord with our strengths and weaknesses and
our virtues and vices. We are learning that for psychological functions terms like "illness" and "health" are analogical, and no more
to be taken literally than are metaphors like "treating" a "sick"
society. We are learning that the concept of "cure," in its purely
medical sense, has outlived its usefulness. And that the prophet,
the priest, the social reformer, the educator and the psychoanalyst
—all those who ask us to change ourselves and the world around
us—have models which are better suited to understanding and
doing something about the vicissitudes of living. Perhaps our most
appropriate models will come from the—unfelicitously named—
social scientists, who, like Freud, destroy our most cherished and
intimate illusions so that we may build more honest and useful
lives. But that remains to be seen.

This book is about halfway houses. The halfway house is
no panacea for all those too psychologically troubled to live in
ordinary society. There is no aim here to present it as such. But
because the halfway house movement is recent, because it took its
impetus from diverse sources, and because halfway houses have as
yet no standardized format—for personnel, for social structure,
for functions and operating procedures—they can serve as field
laboratories for testing different approaches. The tests themselves
are crude. But in the process of examination we can perhaps come
upon some ideas which freshen our vision, extend our scope, and
help us on the way toward a language and a model based on fewer
bad assumptions. Even a small gain in understanding can reverberate in the mitigation of suffering. And that perhaps is enough
for right now. At the bottom of Pandora's box was Hope.

This book began with a demonstration grant (R11-
MH454-03 NIMH) by the National Institute of Mental Health

to Woodley House, a halfway house in Washington, D. C. The grant provided support for a survey of halfway houses. The survey, undertaken by Charlotte Raush, became the basis for a master's thesis submitted to The University of Michigan School of Social Work. It is also the data base from which this book developed. Harold Raush came to know Woodley House through several years of participation on its Board of Trustees and as clinical consultant for a time.

Over the years we learned something about other halfway houses. Particularly, it was meeting with some of those who were directly and intensely involved, as we were not, with day-to-day life in halfway houses which led us to feel that the halfway house movement should be described. And, moreover, that it should be described in sufficient detail to bring out theoretical implications for changes in ways of dealing with the psychologically disturbed and to serve, at the same time, as a practical guide for those who may be interested in starting a halfway house. Our own theoretical biases will not, we would hope, limit the variety of experiments possible within the halfway house framework. That is, what halfway house workers report having learned in practice can be useful apart from the broader implications we have tried to draw.

The dedication to Joan Doniger and Edith Maeda, who run Woodley House, can only suggest the extent to which they inspired this study. Their clearheaded devotion to their tasks of working with highly disturbed people, their willingness to question accustomed tenets, their integrity, independence and their friendship are the sources leading to this point. We are indebted to Leonard Gottesman for his careful reading of the manuscript and for a number of suggestions for improvement; needless to say, he is not responsible for the errors or inadequacies which remain. Virginia Gross' editing improved the clarity of what we tried to say. Much of the labor of preparation of this book was done by Jo-Anna Featherman. In addition to her skills as typist, secretary, researcher, and grammarian, she brought a rare intelligence and devotion to this work; the book owes much to her.

H. L. R.

CONTENTS

Part II

STRUCTURES

Part III

OPERATIONS

Part IV

THE FUTURE OF HALFWAY HOUSES

Part

I

BEGINNINGS

Chapter 1   A LOOK AT THE PAST

PRACTICAL ENDEAVORS OFTEN PRECEDE THEORY AND RESEARCH. A procedure, a technology, a mode of action may exist for many years before it is seen to exemplify a general principle. But when recognition shows us familiar events in a new context, that which we have long ignored emerges to engender new ideas and inventions.

Hardly new, for example, are communal approaches to dealing with mental suffering. More than a thousand years ago the town of Gheel evolved from its beginnings as a seventh century shrine for lunatics into a unique communal colony where those called insane lived in cottages or private homes of the village and its adjacent farming hamlets (Henry, 1941). And Gheel, although probably the oldest historically, was not the sole community developed in an effort to provide those too disturbed to manage in more ordinary societies with a mode of living as social beings. Bockoven (1957) speaks of the late eighteenth century period in New England when, under the sway of the "transcendental" movement, the asylum for the insane was an extension of the physician's household, and the sufferer himself an extension of the physician's family. Charles Dickens, in describing one of these "retreats," tells of the evening lectures and concerts, of the gardening, fishing and hunting, of the availability of horses and carriages for drives

3

in the country (*Action for Mental Health*, 1961). So, too, long before any formal definition, and indeed long before the term itself came into being, halfway houses existed. As early as 1781, there were in England such houses for the "insane poor" (Huseth, 1962).

Although the formal development of halfway houses, as such, is rather recent, numerous informal parallels must have existed for a long time. And unquestionably there are today many informal facilities for mediating between a person with emotional problems and the community with its opportunties and requirements. In any city sufficiently large to have a diversity of boarding homes, there will be found a landlady who prides herself in providing some modicum of community life for those difficult and eccentric isolates, who might be classified psychiatrically as chronic ambulatory schizophrenics; probably there are other landladies who pride themselves on being able to manage "rough" characters and to keep out of trouble those whom psychiatrists would classify as psychopathic personalities or acting-out character neurotics; some landladies, too, no doubt pride themselves on reforming alcoholics, or at least in keeping them sober enough to hold down jobs. Some few boarding homes thus might (or might not) be thought of as halfway houses, though by the definition we shall employ they are not. But that definition is simply a matter of investigative convenience. What is important to recognize is that where there is a social need on the part of some body of people, and where there are those willing to meet this need, a social institution is likely to arise—however informal, however naive, and however inadequate it may be.

Although the term "halfway house" seems to have been used informally before 1953 the earliest definition in the literature appears then in a paper by Reik. Reik comments ". . . that an environment between the hospital and the outside world—a halfway house—would make an important contribution to the rehabilitation of properly selected patients. Having moved from the restricted and dependent existence of the mental hospital to the more independent, but still relatively simple, life at the 'halfway house,' [the ex-patient] would logically be better prepared to take his place in his own community again (p. 616)." Reik describes Spring Lake Ranch in Vermont—which incidentally was founded some twenty years earlier—as exemplifying this definition. In 1954 Rutland Corner House, which had for many years been a temporary home for working women, became a transitional residence for discharged mental patients, thus openly recognizing the need for a specific institution to serve transitional functions (Landy, 1960; Landy & Greenblatt, 1965; Lyman, 1961).

In 1957, Greenblatt and Lidz speak of halfway houses as being relatively rare in America. They mention only one such house, but they describe the halfway house as one of a number of facilities developed in recent years to serve as transitions between the closed mental hospital and the open community. Other intermediate facilities which they mention are day hospitals, night hospitals, sheltered workshops, ex-patient clubs, and family home care programs. The halfway house differs from the others in that it is a somewhat formalized residential institution. Huseth (1962) describes the halfway house as ". . . a residential institution designed to meet needs of the ex-mental patient during the difficult transition from the sheltered environment of the mental hospital to the more rigorous life of the community." All more recent definitions have much the same character, and raise questions we later examine.

In 1960, the *Journal of Social Issues* devoted a special issue to the description of transitional facilities for ex-mental patients. One of the papers, by Henry Wechsler, presents a survey of halfway houses undertaken for the Joint Commission on Mental Illness and Health. Wechsler reports finding seven professionally oriented halfway houses, all of which had been founded since 1954. Distinguished from these were three facilities which Wechsler designates as "work camp houses." Situated in rural settings, they functioned as small communities providing employment and social activities on the grounds rather than in the larger, normal community. Wechsler speaks of the common set of functions which halfway houses share: "On the most obvious level, the halfway house provides a residence for mental patients who no longer need to remain hospitalized but are as yet unable to establish independent residence in the community. Thus the halfway house is intended to serve as a bridge between the hospital and community for patients who either have no home to return to, or whose home is considered to be unsuitable, and who are not yet considered prepared to meet demands and stresses of community life (p. 21)." In the same journal issue Landy (1960) describes Rutland Corner House which since 1954 had been operating as a halfway house.

Some two years later, Ghan (1962) finds thirteen halfway houses in the United States. Ghan does not distinguish between halfway houses and "work camp houses," but he adds four additional settings to Wechsler's list for the United States, and he omits one house which had closed in the interim.

The present survey—again making no sharp distinction between halfway houses and "work camp houses"—found that in the spring of 1963 there were forty settings which could be described formally as halfway houses.

If we look at the founding dates of these forty houses, we discover that only three were established before 1953; five years later there were thirteen established halfway houses. And the present number suggests a further almost four-fold increase in the last five years. It would no doubt be foolish to attempt to extrapolate future development from the rate of growth at this point. But it is clear, both from this growth and from informal comments by participants at a recent conference on halfway houses (Woodley House Conference, 1963) that the movement is still a rapidly expanding one—and that there is as yet no decline in its rate of acceleration.[1]

Professional recognition of this development has also come rather suddenly: the Fifth Volume of the Joint Commission on Mental Illness and Health on *Community Resources in Mental Health* (Robinson, de Marche, & Wagle, 1960) makes no mention of halfway houses. Only a year later, however, in their final report, *Action for Mental Health* (1961), the Commission devotes several

---

[1] Informal estimates suggest that the number of halfway houses in the United States had increased to over 100 by mid-1967.

pages of brief comment to halfway houses, describing (*a*) the cooperative urban house, (*b*) the rural work-oriented halfway house and (*c*) the treatment-oriented halfway facility. By late 1963, Maeda and Rothwell were able to find 144 bibliographic references relating to halfway house programs.

What accounts for the change and what accounts for the sudden and rapid spurt in the movement toward transitional facilities including the halfway house? To understand what has been happening we need to look both at the present situation and at its historical roots.

The major immediate circumstance precipitating the need for transitional facilities was the advent of drug therapies. With the introduction of ataractic drugs, such as chlorpromazine and reserpine, the number of patients in mental hospitals was reduced. In 1954, for the first time in over half a century, there was a drop in the mental hospital population—even though admissions had increased. Further reductions have occurred each year since—always in spite of increased admissions (Klerman, 1961). Few advocates of the drugs claimed that they "cured," and indeed it became apparent that if many of those released were to continue their stay out of the hospital, they had to be maintained on drugs. Still, the discovery of drugs which could, at the least, inhibit the more disrupting aspects of psychopathology made possible the release of large numbers of mental patients, many of whom had been incarcerated for long periods of time. Since the tranquilizing drugs reduced the bizarre symptoms which people in an ordinary community found intolerable, it became feasible for the ex-mental patient to return to the community.

But often for those who had been gone a long time there was no longer a community. One who has been confined to back wards for five years or more can not easily reenter into a family which has by now adjusted to his absence or has extruded and forgotten him (cf. Freeman & Simmons, 1963). And even if a reasonably satisfactory family or living situation exists, long hospitalization will have taken other tolls. One toll is psychological. The long-term patient loses his role as wage earner, as husband, as father. He becomes—often with the encouragement of the hospital—a "patient," with the image of himself as a "patient" (Polansky, White, & Miller, 1957). Another toll is simply that of having been "out of it," of a world changing while he, like Rip van Winkle, has slept. Hospital incarceration offers little education toward coping with the range of problems of living in a typical urban social community, and the rapid rate of present-day social changes exacts an especially high cost from those who have taken a long leave from everyday life. What clearly was called for, then, was the development of new structures to solve these problems of transition and new atmospheres to enhance possibilities for rehabilitation.

These immediate currents coalesced with, colored and were colored by a number of historical influences. Among the influences were: (a) developments in social psychiatry; (b) the impact of psychoanalysis; (c) residential work with children; (d) studies by social scientists; and (e) changing conceptions of "mental illness."

Chapter 2   THE FORCES
            TOWARD INNOVATION

Developments in Social Psychiatry

IF ONE PERSON CAN BE THOUGHT THE FATHER OF SOCIAL PSYCHIATRY, that person is Philippe Pinel (1745–1826). Certainly Pinel had his precursors—in the humanist philosopher Vives and in the physicians Paracelsus, Agrippa, and Johan Weyer, rare isolated voices of rationality in the 16th century world of witches, demons, inquisition and torture (cf. Zilboorg, 1941). But in the more than two hundred years since the dominance of that compendium of witchcraft and source book for inquisitors, the *Malleus Maleficarum*, the lot of the madman had improved only slightly. Although he was no longer tortured as an accomplice of the devil, the victim was interned, chained and fettered with no hope of release. Starved and beaten by keepers, sometimes exhibited as a sadistic source of public entertainment, he was left to rave and to rot in prison-like institutions. One such institution, housing "madmen," was the Bicêtre in Paris. Appointed to the Bicêtre in 1793, in the shadow of the French revolution, Pinel began to remove the chains from those incarcerated there. A short while later he extended his reforms to the six hundred women internees of the madhouse at the Salpêtrière. What was amazing was that the release of these "wild animals" did not have the violent consequences feared by authorities. Rather, once unfettered, the animals became more human. Indeed, Pinel ". . . discovered that insanity was curable, in many instances, by mildness of treatment and attention to the mind exclusively . . . [and that] . . . these principles of moral treatment alone will, frequently, not only lay the foundation of, but complete a cure; while neglect of them may exasperate each succeeding paroxysm, till, at length, the disease becomes established, continued in its form and incurable (Pinel, P. *A Treatise on Insanity,* 1806; quoted in *Action for Mental Health,* 1961, p. 29)."[1]

Pinel thus converted the madhouse to the mental *hospital.* But there was a paradox here. For Pinel rejected the common medical notion of the times that derangement was the result of an organic lesion of the brain and he rejected the medical treatment which was applied to those few who could afford it—the ". . . numerous bloodlettings, cold baths, and violent and repeated showers, with almost no attention paid to *the moral side of the treatment* (Italics Pinel's; Pinel, P. *Traité Medico-philosophique,* 1800; quoted in Zilboorg, 1941, p. 337)." Moreover, Pinel suspected the medical scientificism of his day—the classifications, the magic of words such as diagnosis and prognosis. He speaks of his attempt to view with the eyes of common sense and without prejudice, and there is a modern phenomenological ring to his description. In the PREFACE to his *Traité,* there is a phrase, hardly echoed for more than a hundred years until the advent of Freud, and still in our own times all too fresh: "And how dare we fix the limits which divide what is normal from what borders on a state of illness?"

At the time that Pinel was beginning his great reforms, in 1792, an English Quaker merchant, William Tuke, proposed that the Society of Friends in York found a new institution. Aroused by the abominable conditions in asylums, Tuke established York

---

[1] How "modern" this discovery still is, is suggested by recent studies which indicate that the behavior we have accepted as characteristic of some animals is a function of studying them under conditions of zoo incarceration, and that such behavior in no way resembles that of these animals in their natural environments (Washburn & DeVore, 1961). The study of ecology and behavior is still in its beginning stages (cf. Barker, 1960, 1965).

Retreat. The Retreat, continued under the direction of his children and grandchildren, set an example for humane and reasonable treatment of the deranged.

The institution and Tuke's reforming zeal—his insistence that lunatics were human beings rather than an alien species—had short, but glorious influence in America in the "transcendental" era. We have referred to Dickens' description of one institution so inspired. In commenting on the matter, Dickens adds in his 1842 "Notes": "It is obvious that one great feature of this system is the inculcation and encouragement, even among such unhappy persons, of a decent self-respect (quoted in *Action for Mental Health*, 1961, p. 32)." How cogent these words, and how embarrassingly inapplicable to our present-day institutions. Perhaps, too, it is noteworthy that William Tuke was a layman and that Pinel spoke of his own ideas being initiated through the positive example of a lay superintendent.

Our purpose here is not to trace the history of psychiatry. But clearly the reforms of Pinel and Tuke were not long maintained. With the pressures of urbanization and population growth the asylum became the distant dumping ground for social rejects. The strident notions of popularized Darwinism played a part: the insane suffered from degenerative diseases of the brain; they were the unfit of society, to be cast off in man's evolutionary rise. One could classify, diagnose, prognosticate, but the end result was the same—except for occasional spontaneous remission—incurability and decline. *Moral treatment* was given up. The function of the hospital was the maintenance of the patient and the protection of society. And although keepers were called medical aides or attendants and chains had disappeared, technology simply instituted less weighty restraints. The job of keeper in some social outpost could hardly be expected to attract competent personnel, and the professionals and nonprofessionals who drifted into such work were often hardly less alienated than their charges. It is a sign of the atmosphere of the times that the famed 11th Edition of the Encyclopaedia Britannica (1910) had no entry under *psychiatry* and none under *psychotherapy*.

One great reform had lasted, but it had become a pallid

and empty thing. No longer witches, no longer bestial madmen, the insane were now "sick." But this potentially humane and hopeful term became merely a euphemism. No "sick" people were ever treated as these were, for there was no sickness like this one.

Although there have been periodic pressures and periodic reforms in hospitals since the days of Pinel and Tuke, it was not until the 1950's that a movement arose which could show direct descent from the work of these pioneers. The major impact of this new movement came from a unit established by Maxwell Jones at Belmont Hospital in England. Jones recognized that established hospital practice often bore little relation to treatment needs and that hospital staff often collaborated to erect elaborate defenses for protecting themselves from such needs (Jones, 1953). Working with a population of sociopaths—people who were in trouble because of persistent antisocial behavior, a group commonly recognized as notoriously difficult subjects for psychiatric influence—Jones developed a program which coherently planned and organized activities from morning to night. The formal notion of treatment as consisting of a schedule of appointments with a white-coated doctor was discarded. The treatment agency became the total environment and the total environment was the agency for treatment. Patients stayed at the Unit some two to four months; then active attempts were made to reintegrate them into the general community. Intensive followup and posthospital care was provided by visiting public health nurses. Emergency needs were met with flexibility still radical for mental hospital wards: those needing to reenter the hospital could come in for one night, the weekend, or several days, leaving when they were able.

Jones referred to the Belmont project as a transitional community. In contrast to the usual hospital, which, even if it could boast of an intensive therapy program, was structurally designed as a permanent or semi-permanent station of last resort, the Unit at Belmont was structurally a way station. It was not so much a hospital ward as—in Jones' term—a "therapeutic community."

The notion of "the therapeutic community" has in its short

life been so abused, that it has become attenuated to little more than a popular psychiatric cliche. A change in ward decor, the institution of group therapy, giving patients a vote about television programs—any of these can apparently warrant the title of "therapeutic community." Yet Jones' idea was more than that of making the hospital a pleasant and interesting place to live—a procedure which Jones says might be dysfunctional in that it might entirely fail to prepare for life outside the hospital. The notion thus goes beyond the tolerance and the genteel humaneness of the "moral treatment" era—in theory, if not in practice. Rapaport (1960), who studied the Belmont Unit between 1953 and 1956, speaks of six basic elements as characterizing the therapeutic community (p. 22–23):

1. The total social organization—not just the doctor-patient relation—is seen as affecting therapeutic outcome.

2. The social organization is not simply a background but "a vital force, useful for creating a milieu that will maximize therapeutic effects (p. 22)."

3. The notion includes opportunity for patients to take an active part in the affairs of the institution—democratization in various forms.

4. *All* relationships within the hospital are regarded as potentially therapeutic, including those among the patients themselves.

5. The atmosphere or emotional climate is recognized as important.

6. Communication *per se* is highly valued.

The fundamental idea is an overt commitment to the position that everything is grist for the treatment mill, and the presumed consequence is that all aspects of the patients' lives become subject to analysis and intervention. Rapaport (1960) comments that "interventions on any of the recognized levels (sociocultural, psychological, biological) may be used to yield results on other levels (p. 27)."

Despite these radical innovations, Jones' procedures were still in many ways those of the hospital. Jones speaks of the Belmont Project as involving a "unit of one hundred beds." The residents are "patients"; to leave the hospital, they must get "passes"; bedtime is fixed at 9:00. Jones describes how, in contrast to the practice of the rest of the Hospital, doctors and nurses share tables in the dining room. But both groups eat apart from the patients. Rapaport notes the discrepancies between the informal role conceptions encouraged by the Unit and the formal ones within professions and within the Hospital, and he notes the staff role conflicts. Moreover, he suggests that there is often a divergence and conflict between the activities and designs appropriate to treatment—that is, "the reorganization of individual dynamics," and those appropriate to rehabilitation—that is, "the adjustment of the individual to his social role." The goals of social adaptation and those of personality change must, Rapaport believes, be distinguished from each other, for the procedures under one goal can be incompatible with those under the other.

Rapaport's distinction is an attempt to make sense of a confused conceptual system. The "therapeutic community" was a response to the inadequacy of a medical model of specific focused "treatment" for the specific "illnesses" of "patients." The model had broken down because it was too rigid. A sociopsychological scheme of function and malfunction was grafted onto the medical model, but the graft did not quite take. At Belmont there were signs on the walls with cartoons of patients at workshops, at play, dancing and talking. Under each picture was the caption, "This is treatment (Rapaport, 1960, p. 52)." One might well respond, "*This* is treatment?" Where "everything is treatment," the notion of "treatment" becomes absurd.

Since the days when Jones initiated the Belmont Unit there have been many other experiments within the hospital model. Hamburg, for example, describes a program for the psychiatric section of a general hospital (Hamburg, 1957). He recognizes that psychiatric patients are not like other hospital patients, and that general hospital administrative policies, with emphasis on objectivity and uniformity, with minimal activity, minimal information and an impersonal atmosphere in relation to patients, are not suitable for a psychiatric section. He suggests modes for facilitating communication between patients and staff and for broadening patient participation in decision making. Similarly, Wilmer (1957, 1958) presents a program which makes heavy use of group methods and which concentrates on issues of communication among neurotic and psychotic patients.

The Cummings, a team of psychiatrist husband and sociologist wife, have had intensive experience in both the United States and Canada in undertaking the major reorganization of mental hospitals (1957). In a recent volume, *Ego and Milieu* (1962), they describe their programs of environmental therapy. Drawing their theories from both sociology and psychiatry, they present a highly explicit approach to milieu therapy. In contrast to psychotherapy which "sets out to make 'basic'—that is, intrapsychic —changes, usually expecting social improvement to follow," they suggest that "milieu therapy sets out to make social changes and trusts that ego growth will ensue (Cumming & Cumming, 1962, p. 271)." They define the therapeutic milieu as a scientific manipulation of the environment aimed at producing changes in the patient. Even crises are manipulated and controlled. The authors suggest that crisis resolution ". . . *should be a therapeutic tool that can be scientifically controlled* (their italics). Thus, if an individual has been unable to solve problems because of inadequate biological endowment or extreme environmental stress, he should experience ego growth and reorganization if he is introduced to carefully controlled minor crises in a protected situation (Cumming & Cumming, 1962, p. 56)." In contrast to usual psychiatric practice, with its verbal emphasis, the emphasis here is on action. And the environment, including lines of administrative authority and lines of communication, is explicitly contrived to promote and induce favorable actions.

The Cummings apply the sociological findings—including their own—of studies of hospitals. But their orientation is clearly and fundamentally a medical one. The assumptive context—that of a hospital, of wards, of physicians, nurses and attendants having clear role definitions, and of formal, explicit hospital rules and proscriptions—is questioned far less than in, for example, Jones' Unit. The ethics of social manipulation—a problem which the Cummings are aware of—is clearly one of medical responsibility; the physician must often define what is best for the patient. Moreover, since the Cummings' definition of a therapeutic milieu requires the notion of controlled manipulation of the environment, they doubt that such a milieu can be created outside a hospital. The kind of precise planning and clarity of boundaries which they recommend could, in their opinion, hardly be achieved in any more "natural" setting. Even the recommendation for hospitals to institute more home-like furnishings and surroundings is made as a rational medical prescription. And since mental hospitals are concerned with masses of patients and with treatment of diseases— rather than with idiosyncrasies of persons—the prescriptions tend to become de-individualized.

A more radically innovative program for the reform of mental hospitals and for the rehabilitation of the severely disturbed is that of Paul Sivadon. Sivadon's work, first at a hospital at Neuilly-sur-Marne and later at le Mesnil Saint-Denis in the environs of Paris, is all too little known, for he has published little in English (1957). Sivadon, a French psychiatrist, speaks of his approach as sociotherapy. In its emphasis on the total milieu, on action, and on attention to processes of communication, his program has much in common with those of Jones and the Cummings. But its scope encompasses more, its theoretical orientation differs, and its model deviates more broadly from one based on illness.

Like that of the Cummings, Sivadon's program is a rational one, in which each of the specifics is carefully thought through and planned in terms of a goal of resocialization. But Sivadon emphasizes heterogeneity and the diversity of arrangements necessary for particular individuals and for particular stages of disturbance. All aspects of living enter into these considerations. Thus, major architecture arrangements are coordinated with individual levels of disturbance. A complex of buildings for those who are most disoriented needs to be a symmetrical array, so that the patient is not made too anxious; when he is improved, the complex of buildings should be asymmetrical so as to offer him a mild challenge. Similarly, the living units must allow for diversity —by building from small units which can be expanded as particular circumstances and particular needs suggest to a series of larger units—so that the patient can increase or decrease his social group easily. In place of homogeneous groupings, groups are balanced so as to provide the potentials for varied relations—mixing ages, sexes, and symptom categories. Sivadon states: "A good therapeutic community should offer to the patient an opportunity to enter into whatever kind of group suits his condition, whether the group be large or small, homogeneous or heterogeneous (1957, p. 206)."

The specific procedures which Sivadon uses for reeducation are, like the architectural notions, geared to concepts of developmental progression. Space and social contact are especially important in this conceptualization. One approach, for example, is through ball play. For the very regressed patient the program starts with the instructor and patient tossing a ball back and forth within a closely confined space. Gradually the distance is increased. "Then a second patient and a third are introduced. Finally, the play is complicated by modifying the position and number of patients, by introducing a second ball, and by interposing first an obstacle, later a screen, between the patient and the instructor (Sivadon, 1957, p. 208)." The same notion of progressive differentiation is put to work in activities such as modeling or painting —the use of tools following a variable period of undifferentiated direct contact with the materials themselves. A series of physical exercises are similarly graded, though active two-person physical contacts, to multi-person complex, asymmetrical, integrated arrangements.

All of Sivadon's procedures are within a context of utmost respect for the individuality of the person. The extent of this consideration is seen in Sivadon's description of how a patient is admitted to the community:

In my service I have had for the past 10 years a psychologist who functions as a hostess to welcome each new patient. She is the first person with whom the patient comes in contact. Instead of taking away his personal effects she gives him whatever he needs—toilet articles, cigarettes, writing paper, and so on. She introduces him to his fellow patients, to his attendants, nurses, and doctors. She tries immediately to make him feel that he was expected and that he is needed—that his help is needed, perhaps, with a party that is being prepared, with a game, or with some little service which no one else can render, such as repairing a bell or a broken chair. Then she shows him around the grounds and buildings, the workshops, the reception rooms, the bar, and the hairdressing parlor. Very quickly, often by joining in a game, the patient makes the acquaintance of two or three comrades with whom he will soon work in the shops. The welcome is rounded out by introducing the patient at the weekly meeting of the committee of patients, of which I shall speak later.

Finally, each week there is a friendly gathering at which the medical director and the hostess meet with the patients who have been admitted in the past seven days. The medical director and hostess find out whether they are provided with everything they need and solicit their criticisms and their ideas. Then each one is given a brochure with his own name printed on it, in which he finds, following some words of welcome, the principal kinds of information which are likely to relieve his anxieties. In particular, he finds there the name of his personal physician and of his social worker. He is also given some visiting cards with which he can introduce himself to his comrades and which he can place at the head of his bed or at the entrance of his cubicle.

Techniques of welcome such as these turn out to be of considerable importance in promoting the rapid participation of the new arrival in the community. In effect, the more one wishes the patient to allow himself to slip quietly into the communal life in a relaxed way, the more important it is to individualize him as much as possible and to make him feel himself to be a person. It is for this reason— namely, to counterbalance the communitarian atmosphere into which he is plunged—that the patient is at first seen privately by his personal physician, who gives him an appointment by a written personal invitation (1957, pp. 206–207).

The mode is, of course, French—for example, the visiting cards. But the rationality, the simple, yet thoughtful humaneness, the individualized attention to personal detail, could well be emulated in any of our own institutions.

Sivadon does not speak of the intellectual roots of his approach, though surely they go back in part to Pinel. But it is important to note that, unlike most conceptualizations in hospital social psychiatry, Sivadon's have a developmental emphasis. Each procedure is premised on notions of developmental stages—proceeding from simple to complex, from undifferentiated to differentiated, from unorganized to integrated, from passive to active control, from symmetry to asymmetry. The conceptual base seems particularly close to Piaget's ideas about cognitive and perceptual development in children (cf. Flavell, 1963), and the procedures are compatible with psychoanalytic ways of looking at the genesis of relationships (cf. Erikson, 1950).

Sivadon does not consciously reject a medical view—he speaks of patients and treatment—but in practice his model is less that of a hospital than of a school. The residents are not so much treated as reeducated. And although it is modish to speak of the rehabilitation of the psychologically alienated as reeducation, Sivadon's work represents more than a fashionable rephrasing and more than the adaptation of a few practical techniques. It is, in contrast with most rehabilitative hospital procedures, securely grounded in a developmental orientation. This grounding, together with the individualized concern and respect accorded to the clientele, creates of Sivadon's institution a unique model—somewhere between a very special boarding school and a well run hotel.

Apart from influencing changes in the structure and program of mental hospitals, developments in social psychiatry have exerted effects on professional modes of responding to the problems of severe psychological disturbance in another way. Increasingly, psychiatrists have become involved in issues of normative developmental crises. They have studied possibilities for helping people through the crisis of mourning (Lindemann, 1944), for alleviating the stress in urban renewal programs (Lindemann, 1960), for socializing the socially outcast (Fishman, Pearl, & MacLennan, 1965), for planning of cities (Duhl, 1963), for consulting with teachers (Caplan, 1956), for easing the problems of separation of the child entering school (Goodrich, 1961), etc. Under these circumstances, the psychiatrist can no longer speak of patients and of illness. His competence and his contribution is in understanding both adverse and favorable modes of coping with the events which are presented to us or which we create. His concern must be with the problems of living in a world of oneself, of other beings, of objects and of organizations, institutions and cultures. Although he speaks of prevention, this is an anachronism of language. His concern is less for the prevention of a hypothetical disease than for a more rational, less painful—or if painful, less uselessly painful —human existence. And although the effects of these developments on the vicissitudes of dealing with the severely disturbed are indirect, they are in the long run likely to be deeper.

The Impact of Psychoanalysis

The historical roots of medicine are in its response to the universal call for the alleviation of suffering. But as the boundaries of suffering move out from the interior milieu of the body to the regions of man's relation with man and to his relation with social institutions, the traditional approaches of medicine become progressively strained. So it was that Freud found himself forced away from the physicalistic biases of the psychiatry of his time. This course was indeed no easy choice for him. One has only to look at his early efforts to establish and maintain a physical rationale for psychological symptoms: his preoccupation with the pseudo-chemical theories of his friend Fliess (Jones, E., 1953; Freud, 1954), or his later attempt to attribute the primary cause of anxiety to the blocking of the physical orgasm. Even when, after relinquishing a physical orientation, he embraced the notion of specific psychological trauma as causing the disturbances which he set himself to cure, he again suffered disappointment. The childhood events related by his patients had often, he found, never actually happened. Increasingly, despite his training and disposition, his observations led him to psychology. And although he never quite gave up hope for the eventual discovery of chemical foundations underlying the profounder mental disturbances, the revolution he created was in his unequivocal view of man as a psychological being.

Freud certainly made no pretense to a full understanding of the severe disturbances, the psychoses, or as he called them, the narcissistic neuroses. Nor did he reject ideas that genetic or chemical factors might contribute to the etiology of psychological disorders or that chemical means might eventually be found for mitigating psychological disturbances. These considerations, however, in no way lessened his convictions as to the psychological relevance of disturbed behavior. Mental suffering was to be understood in psychological, not physical terms. Phenomena senseless in physical terms made sense psychologically.

It is fashionable these days to criticize Freud for a bias toward physicalism, for ignoring man's culture and social environment, for neglect of the interpersonal, and for emphasis on the pathological. Such critiques carry enough truth to germinate the founding of new theories and movements. But none of these criticisms is wholly legitimate and most contemporary movements which emphasize a psychological approach to the amelioration of mental suffering are constructed on one or another cornerstone of the architectural foundation created by Freud.

At the base of psychoanalysis was Freud's insistence that there was always a kind of sense in what people felt and did. However seemingly nonsensical, however bizarre, behavior was not a random epiphenomenon of disordered neural circuits. Actions were meaningful in terms of the premises of the actor. The premises came from memories and distortions of memories, the residues of the culture in which the child was raised. The capacity for suffering from memories was part of the human condition. The premises, going back to origins in childhood, formed templates through which current realities were screened, sieved, and compared. Once and for all, the seeming arbitrariness of behavior was given coherence.

How then does one "cure" memories? The point is that one does not "cure" memories, in any ordinary sense of the word *cure*. One can come to recognize, reorganize, de-emphasize ("decathect") memories, and perhaps even to forget that which once was but no longer is relevant. So in his "treatment" Freud was led ever farther away from the paraphernalia of medicine, discarding the clinic atmosphere of Charcot, resigning the costume and authority of the physician, step by step abjuring the magic of physical methods, of hypnosis, of suggestion. With the method of free association, patient and therapist became co-participant explorers. A major aspect of the "cure" concerned the relation between the two, a relation peculiarly structured to allow fullest explorations of past interpersonal relations through study of their current effects. "Cure" was through understanding—psychological understanding.

If even the strangest behavior had meaning, it could be understood, and hopefully that understanding could be used in effecting changes. But there was yet another aspect of the psychoanalytic viewpoint which had profound influence on the position of the mentally disturbed. This was the general dynamic theory of the unconscious, a theory of forces and counter-forces. The specifics of the theory need not concern us here. What is relevant is that the general theory of psychic function was applicable to both so-called "normal" and "abnormal" phenomena. There was but one psychopathology. The "normal" person did not escape from it. It appeared in his dreams, his humor, his slips of the tongue, and in his sometimes serious lapses from rationality. In an attenuated and usually somewhat controlled form, he showed the "abnormalities" which were exaggerated in the more severely disturbed. The history he bore was a somewhat happier version of equivalent events. We were all, patient and nonpatient, as Harry Stack Sullivan later put it, "more simply human than otherwise."

The patient in the mental hospital was thus rescued—if only theoretically—from his position as member of a strange and alien species. His mental processes and his actions, although difficult to fathom, were essentially no less comprehensible than our own. Psychoanalysis offered a theory and a method for this understanding. More than these, it offered a hope.

The influence of psychoanalysis on those confined in mental hospitals was slow to be felt. On the one hand, the hope started a surge of activity and humane concern such as had not been seen since the early days of "moral" treatment. The impetus was most sharply felt following the Second World War with the massive increase in demands for psychiatric service and increase in training for mental health workers. The new young psychiatrists, psychologists and social workers were strongly influenced by the scope, breadth and power of understanding offered by psychoanalysis. They were inspired by the pioneering efforts of the few devoting themselves to the herculean rescue of those humans who seemed beyond human reach. The work of Paul Federn, Frieda Fromm-Reichmann, Robert Knight, John Rosen, and Harry Stack Sullivan was eagerly absorbed. Although the theories of these pioneers differed, all were psychoanalytic at the core. All offered a path for work and for the adventure of human understanding.

Failure of the new hope to become a social force in modifying the lot of the hospitalized lay less in the inadequacies of psychoanalytic theory (though it is partly there) than in the demands of the psychoanalytic method. Psychoanalysis evolved for those who were capable—by virtue of their articulateness, their awareness, their capacity for control, their economic and social stability—of meeting the psychological, social and economic demands imposed by psychoanalytic treatment. For the severely disturbed, as for children, the treatment model required modification. This Freud clearly recognized, as did every psychoanalytic worker after him. But which parameters of treatment (Eissler, 1953) to modify and how to modify them have never received any fully satisfying answer.

The second basis for failure of psychoanalysis as a social force in dealing with the severely disturbed lay in the demands psychoanalysis makes on the practitioner. The requirements for training of psychoanalysts—and indeed, for training of any form of capable therapist—make it unlikely that there will ever be a sufficient number of practitioners to meet social demands. "In sum, then," to quote *Action for Mental Health*, "psychoanalysis is adapted neither to the treatment of the psychoses nor to mass application of any kind (1961, p. 80)." Of course, acknowledgement that the specific method cannot be applied directly or en masse negates neither the contributions of the theory nor its social implications.

The major influence of psychoanalysis on social approaches —such as the halfway house—to working with the psychologically alienated is in its emphasis on the unity of psychological suffering and in its focus on psychological determination. Psychoanalysis brought into scrutiny the reality of the psyche. Perhaps because the implications of such scrutiny were so massive, it gave little attention to the analysis of social reality. Yet the social situation, if not adequately emphasized by psychoanalysis, was not wholly neglected. Even in rather early writings (Freud, 1900), Freud described how actual experiences from the previous day (day-residues) influenced and helped form the dreams one had that night. The social situation received a similar, if secondary, focus in relation to psychopathology. Through its connection with previous memory traces, the current situation was seen as providing precipitating circumstances for the formation of symptoms. And in one of his last papers, *Analysis Terminable and Interminable* (1937), Freud gave explicit consideration to the limitations of psychoanalysis as related to environmental and other life circumstances. Moreover, present day psychoanalytic thought, particularly as exemplified by Erikson (1950, 1959), devotes considerable effort to exploring the relations of the social demands and opportunities in particular societies to individual patterns of personal development. It is in these latter explorations that the hope of such approaches as represented by the halfway house have their theoretical base.

Residential Work with Children

It is hard to be sure whether or not influences from residential work with children have had any *direct* impact on the halfway house movement. Some founders and directors of halfway houses have, like those at Woodley House, come to their work only after extensive experience in children's residential settings; many with no direct experience nevertheless express ideas which parallel the views of those who have thought most about working with disturbed children within a residential milieu. Whether or not a direct line of influence exists, comparing issues in the treatment of disturbed adults and children is useful, for work with children highlights problems and, in a few instances, faces them more squarely.

Consider first the hospital. The primary task of the hospital is to cure or at least minister to the suffering of sick patients. Ideally, all other tasks are subsidiary and geared to this main aim. Care-taking is important, since it is instrumental to the primary medical goal, but nonetheless it is auxiliary to that goal. Since people coming to the usual hospital are most often seriously ill, care-taking functions must be tailored to the needs of the bed-ridden patient. And these functions must be organized for efficiency and so as to enhance and in no way interfere with medical requirements. The system of wards and stations, each for patients having similar illnesses, the centralization of cooking, laundry and purchasing, the hierarchy of differentiated responsibility in physicians, nurses, and attendants, accomplishes this organization. So, too, do the professional training and the inculcated culture and lore which enter into creating and maintaining a hospital atmosphere. Thus, for example—at least up until very recently—efforts are made to project an anonymity onto the patient, and staff are warned off close personal involvement with patients. The patient is a "case," a collection of diseased organs, because the lore is—not without justification—that any other view would interfere with the primary task of cure.

Even today, in this country, most children's psychiatric facilities are organized along those familiar hospital lines. But because even the most psychologically maladapted children are active and growing beings, they help pinpoint the dilemmas of usual psychiatric hospital structure and practice. For example, it is apparent that if children are ever to enter into an everyday ordinary world, not only must their physical needs be met, but also they must encounter educational and social experiences relevant to their society. The tasks and experiences of growing up cannot simply be postponed for the time required for a specific therapeutic procedure.

For one thing, the work of growing up and the experiences which may either inhibit this work or make it possible are central to the disturbed child's difficulties, and so cannot be bypassed. Second, it is more apparent with children than with adults that the absence of some experiences does not constitute simply an isolated blank—that something goes on that reverberates on other experience and that sets a course for future experience. Lack of experience with peers, or with family roles, or with learning to read or write, or with affection or with accomplishment is not simply a localized emptiness, but is substituted for in fantasy, attitude or activity and casts a shadow far into the future. Third, work with children makes it apparent that they are less capable of the differentiations generally expected of adults. This is true of young, normal children (Werner, 1957; Flavell, 1963), and disturbed children are even less able to establish and maintain differentiations. In severe pathology, boundaries and differentiations seem not to exist. Each event, each sphere of experience tends to fuse with past events into the next event and experience. Those who have worked in residential children's settings know that a poorly selected game or a bad school hour strikingly and immediately influences the adjacent psychotherapy hour; and they see a difficulty in a psychotherapy hour reverberate to a temper tantrum in school or a fight in a peer interaction.

There has been much confusion in the use of the term "therapeutic milieu," and the term, like "therapeutic community," has come to be little more than a shibboleth whereby one indicates that he is in tune with the times in an awareness that the therapy hour is not all, that there is a world which has impact on the patient for good or for ill. But as originally used by Redl and Wineman (1951, 1952) and by Bettelheim (1950) the use of the term "therapeutic milieu" implied that in the treatment of disturbed children the immediate environment was a major influence; that for even normal children to develop, environments must provide essential features, graded in terms of the child's stage of development; and furthermore, that with disturbed children, environments could and needed to be planned in relation to the child's disturbance. Within a treatment institution, influence emanates not only from the ascribed therapy authorities—psychiatrists, psychologists or social workers—but from all those whose work impinges on the child, whether or not their intentions are directly "therapeutic"—teachers, attendants, maids and cooks.

Not only do the people in the environment make a difference; objects and their arrangement are important. As Redl notes, long hallways suggest running, and elevator buttons on walls ask to be pushed. Too few and too familiar play objects fail to stimulate the child. Too many and too new objects can be overstimulating—as parents of even "normal" young children learn at Christmas. The bright deprived child will need more objects in his environment; the dull, brain-damaged child will need fewer. Object arrangements and architecture may crowd, isolate, cheer, depress, simplify, complicate, challenge, bore, delight or repulse, welcome or frighten.

Those who pioneered in residential work with disturbed children—in this country, Bruno Bettelheim and Fritz Redl particularly—have thus found it necessary, if they are to be effective in modifying severe pathology, to encompass in their programs the entire range of experiences a child undergoes. Their work suggests that no part of the highly disturbed child's life space can be casually ignored. Bettelheim, working predominantly with schizophrenic children in residential treatment, showed that psychotherapy could not be isolated from the social milieu in which the child was treated, and that intensive planning of the total environment was necessary in working with these very disturbed children. Redl and Wineman, in residential work with very aggressive children, presented explicit and dramatic details on the sensitivities of such children to milieu factors, and they separated the factors which were destructive from those conducive to the progress of the children.

Architectural arrangements, group size and heterogeneity, the personal characteristics of staff, the scheduling and availability of food, the timing and character of games, the structure and size of a classroom, the distribution of clothes, toys, pocket money— all offer opportunities for constructive or destructive outcomes. Neither simple satisfaction of physical needs nor simple good will are enough. Plans and arrangements must be geared to the developmental saliency of particular experiences. And that requires knowledge both of general developmental issues relevant to a particular age and sex and of specific developmental issues relevant for a particular child (Redl, 1959b).

To the extent that workers become aware of the above issues, residential treatment tends to deviate from the hospital model. The new model often comes closer to that of a very special boarding school or a very special children's camp. Seldom does it become that of a family home.[2]

Few psychiatric hospitals have broken with the hospital tradition and with the requisites posed by the hospital model. Sivadon's hospital perhaps comes closest to attempting innovations somewhat like those tried in the residential treatment of children. In general, the relevance of and need for alternative models in dealing with problems of severe psychological maladaptation have

[2] The claim of being modeled on the family is most often made by those in traditional hospital settings; its absurdity is apparent in the ward structure, in the number of children, in the three daily shifts of workers. There are some children's institutions in Norway and Sweden which come close to exemplifying a home model. Children are in cottages of no more than six; the age and sex grouping in a cottage may be heterogeneous; the primary staffing is by a couple who live in the cottage; and it is these arrangements which are combined with intensive professional and nonprofessional services. Indicative of how much like home these cottages are was an answer given to the query: "How do you convince your legislators and the public to pay the high cost of these arrangements?" The answer was something like this: "It isn't at all hard to convince people about this. Everyone knows how difficult and expensive it is to raise a normal family of six children. When we tell them about our kind of children it is obvious to people that the needs are much greater."

been more difficult to perceive for adults than for children. But, as we see, it is the search for alternative models, better geared to a recognition of psychological need and environmental opportunity, which has, wittingly or unwittingly, moved the initiators of halfway houses.

Studies by Social Scientists

The halfway house stands on a vague border between the person—usually a mental hospital patient recently discharged—and the community. If we may for a moment separate the clinical sciences, such as psychiatry and clinical psychology, from the social sciences, we find the borderland between person and community has generally been the purview of the more socially oriented scientists. Thus it is that the major theoretical and empirical contributions to the development of the halfway house movement have come from sociologists, social psychologists, anthropologists, and—certainly in practice if not so much in theory—social workers. Once again, the impact is not necessarily direct; it may often be a secondary *geist* seeping into the body of lore of such diverse fields as nursing, occupational therapy, education and vocational rehabilitation. Some of the influence—which for the sake of simplicity we identify as sociological—has already been suggested in the section on Social Psychiatry.

Since Durkheim, modern sociology has been interested in the relations between the social order and personal deviance. The tradition of interest has spread in several directions. On the one hand are broad-scale, rather epidemiological studies, relating incidence and prevalence of psychopathology to social factors. A classic early example is the work of Faris and Dunham (1939) who plotted the prevalence of mental disorder in relation to social demarcations of urban Chicago. A modern example appears in the work of Hollingshead and Redlich (1958), a sociologist and a psychiatrist, respectively, who demonstrated the major effects of a person's socio-economic class background on the likelihood of his obtaining professional psychological help and on what happens to him if he is severely deviant. Branching from this direction are studies which attempt to relate more specific facts of personality (Miller & Swanson, 1958) and child-rearing practices (Kohn, 1959) to social class factors. A second direction has taken the form of surveys by social psychologists of attitudes toward deviance, toward mental health professions, or toward seeking and receiving help for psychological problems (Gurin, Veroff, & Feld, 1960). Studies in either of these directions have helped broaden the base of thinking about issues of psychological deviance. They have pointed beyond the problems of intrapsychic conflict, and they have indicated that such problems derive their particular relevance and their particular solutions in relation to the social order. They thus are important for the halfway house, concerned with integration between the person and the social community.

Still a third direction of sociological work concerns us primarily here. As already suggested, a main motive for the development of halfway houses arises from the limitations imposed by hospital structure. Sociological research and thinking have been the prime movers in focusing awareness on the patterns of social interaction inherent in particular institutional arrangements. In the 1950's the mental hospital was subjected to a number of such critical appraisals.

A major impact on psychiatric thought was the result of a collaborative effort between a psychiatrist and a sociologist. In 1954, Alfred Stanton and Morris Schwartz described the mental hospital as a community. They illustrated how the structure, functions and problems of this community influenced and modified the behavior of those who came to the hospital for treatment. Stanton and Schwartz were able, for example, to relate the ebb and flow of symptomatology among patients to the prevalence or absence of communication difficulties among staff. Intra-staff conflict and poor communication, whether or not patients were aware of these, were reflected in the exacerbation of disturbed patient behavior. That is, they found that an interference in communication between two staff members, each of whom was in contact with a patient but who were in *covert* disagreement about the patient's management, was regularly accompanied by pathological excitement on the part of the patient. Role confusions among staff were reflected in the patient's confusion.

Independently, William Caudill, a social anthropologist, described the mental hospital as a small society (Caudill, 1958; Caudill & Stainbrook, 1954). Caudill, too, was impressed with the effects of covert communication difficulties. He emphasized the separate social worlds of patients and staff, the lack of adequate channels between the worlds, and the development of separate cultures in the two groups.

Perhaps the most telling commentary is that presented by Erving Goffman (1961) in a series of essays which describe the mental hospital as one among a number of "total institutions," such as prisons, monasteries, and military services. A total institution is one which assumes complete authority and control over all aspects of the individual's life, and despite their diverse philosophies and purposes, all such institutions have much in common. For example, the novice on entering is subject to rites of stripping and mortification; he must give up his ordinary clothes, his ordinary habits, and all those features which mark individuality in usual social life. He loses all former rank, status, and distinction, and becomes part of a depersonal, anonymous uniformity.[3] The institution has its own culture, one not open to outsiders, and all participants share in the inside-outside differentiation and in a common body of lore.

But within the institution itself there are two cultures—that of staff and that of inmates. Staff is responsible for all aspects of the inmate's life. Staff is organized into a hierarchy which the inmate understands only vaguely; nevertheless he is subject to control by any staff member. The sanctions by which control is exercised are unlike those of usual society. For example, in ordinary society an argument with one's boss may result in restrictions in one's work situation; it does not connect directly with restrictions in one's social life. In contrast, within a total institution such

---

[3] We have referred to Sivadon's efforts to counter this process.

as a mental hospital, behavior in one sphere of life directly affects every other sphere; the patient who blows up at the lunch table may be kept from participating in sports the next day. Staff exercises control through a system of "privileges." What are called "privileges" in total institutions are the "rights" of ordinary society—to shave oneself, to smoke, to come and go freely when one is not under a mutually entered contractual arrangement.[4] Staff develops a code of administration and of administrative distance. Emphasis is on the "good," quiet, efficient ward, the absence of personality and its messiness, the difference between inmate and staff.

Inmates develop their own culture, sometimes with an institutional language and signs known only to initiates. An internal code of how to get by is part of this culture, and the wise inmate—sometimes after a period of initial rebellion or withdrawal —will learn how to play it cool and con the system. Goffman also describes the rituals, the institutional newspaper, and the ceremonies, such as the annual party and the theatrical parody, which serve as "role-releases."

A novel by Ken Kesey (1962), illustrates, though it romanticizes, the gaps described by Goffman between the patient and the staff cultures of a mental hospital. The patient who does not "improve," in the sense of becoming "good," affronts the staff. His privileges are removed; he gets less rather than more help; punishment is euphemized as "treatment." The contrast between treatment of the physically ill in the usual hospital and treatment of the deranged in the mental hospital is one that is apparent to even a casual visitor.

Some of the structural bases for complexity and confusion in relations within the mental hospital were noted in 1954 by Jules Henry (Henry, 1954, 1957). Henry described four types of organizational structure. Patterns of *simple subordination* may be *undifferentiated* if the task is treated as a single unit, as in the case of a small shop where everyone performs all functions; or

---

[4] A point Goffman does not emphasize but which is characteristic of the total institution is segregation by sex, and deprivation of normal sexual life.

they may be *differentiated*, as in the case of a supermarket, where the tasks are divided into a number of subunits, with each part in the hands of a different person. In either of the simple subordination structures, however, one person is responsible for direction, and there is one immediate superior from whom a given worker receives orders and to whom he is responsible.

In contrast, hospitals are structured in patterns of *multiple* subordination. In such patterns, lines of responsibility are diffuse. The nurse, for example, theoretically takes orders from any staff doctor, in addition to those from nursing supervisors; attendants are subject to the orders of any nurse and any doctor; and patients, if we include them in the system, are subject to the orders of all nurses, doctors and attendants. The multiple subordination structure may be *differentiated*, as when different aspects of the patient's life become the responsibility of different personnel—for example, occupational therapists, social workers, psychotherapists; or it may be *undifferentiated*, as in the case of the nurse who takes similar orders from five different doctors.

Henry notes that, with the many possibilities for conflicting orders, there are inherent difficulties in multiple subordination, and he suggests that because of the inefficiency in multiple subordination, systems tend to move toward the simple structure. Still it is likely that where tasks are easily divisible and relatively clearcut, as in the case of the general hospital, a structural pattern of multiple differentiated subordination is tenable. The problem is considerably more acute in the mental hospital, where the nature of the patient's problems require that he be treated as a single, total, integrated unit. An additional stress becomes then the tension between the division of labor prescribed in the differentiated pattern and the holistic approach suggestive of an undifferentiated system.

The ambiguities are perhaps most sharply reflected in the role of the psychiatric nurse. Trained for specific nursing duties, she finds herself shorn of medical techniques, and in a vague role of both general manager and general factotum. The ambiguity is reflected in the fact that, although she considers her relations with patients to be therapeutic, the patients themselves do not consider this to be so (Caudill, 1958). It is no wonder then that nurses are prone to quit psychiatric wards in order to go back to "real" nursing. Even the psychiatrist, trained to view his patients holistically, finds himself caught in ambiguous part roles.

Confusions arise not only from structural problems, but also from ambiguities about the functions of the mental hospital. The primary task of the ordinary hospital is to cure.[5] But the task of the psychiatric hospital has never been that clearly defined. At one time the deviant was the direct responsibility of the community, and the community, whether of one family or several, undertook measures, human or inhumane, for custody of the deviant and for needed protection of other members of the community. But with increased urbanization and the attendant age of specialization, which included the development of specialists in mind and behavior, responsibility of the deviant was increasingly delegated by the community to the specialist.

It thus came about that the mental hospital has not one primary task, but rather the four ascribed to it by Parsons (1957): (a) custody of the deviant; (b) protection of the community; (c) socialization of the deviant; and (d) therapy. It is inevitable that these goals conflict with one another. Hospital administrators must, for example, continually weigh decisions which might benefit a particular patient but which might constitute a risk to the protection of the community. Because it is the community which controls the purse strings, the decision is usually on the safe side. Other aims may also conflict. We have previously noted Rapaport's (1960) comments on the divergence and conflict at Belmont between goals of treatment and goals of socialization. Different staff members identify themselves with and give major emphasis to different goals. Attendants tend to see patient needs in terms of custodial care—food, clothing, etc.; rehabilitation workers, occupational therapists and recreation leaders see the primary goal as

---

[5] In historically recent times hospitals have also become places in which to be born and in which to die. Fulfilling these roles no doubt also strains a structure premised on a primary task of cure.

socialization; the higher professional echelons consider therapy to be the hospital's basic task; and administrative directors, as suggested, all too often focus on the protection of the community.

Such considerations have led increasingly to questions of whether hospitals for the psychologically disturbed do more harm than good. Polansky, White & Miller (1957) deplore the extended loss of roles—as wage earner, husband, father—which the psychiatric patient must undergo, and they see as dysfunctional the requirement that he become a "patient" with the "image" of himself as a "patient." Kennard (1957) describes how administrative demands, staff turnover, budgetary factors and bed space become the major determinants of the patient's movement—whether he enters or leaves the hospital and whether he is transferred from one ward to another. Kennard suggests that psychiatric training has little to do with such work. As for the patient, he is mostly a passive subject of these maneuvers, spending most of his time in the day-room. The rebellion, the withdrawal and apathy, the learning to play it cool induced by the system has been the subject of every biographical or novelistic treatment of the mental hospital since Clifford Beers description in 1921. Supporting evidence for the damaging impact of such experience comes from studies dealing with social deprivation and with limitation of psychological input and action (cf. Thibault & Kelley, 1959).

It is no surprise then that Galioni, Notman, Stanton,& Williams, (1957) ask the questions: are wards necessary?; is it necessary to take patients "off the ward" for their "dose" of treatment—occupational, industrial, psycho-, recreational or biblio-therapy—then take them back for cold storage?. They imply that grafting the concept of "cure" onto the concept of custodial "care" has produced a monster.

The viability of the hospital as a model for dealing with major psychological disturbance has thus come under severe question. So long as problems of psychological disability were seen as an issue solely between the "diseased" person and his doctor, other aspects of the environment were auxiliary. It might, of course, be easier to treat the person in a hospital than at home, nurses might be needed to insure proper treatment, exercises might be valuable in avoiding secondary complications, and other auxiliary personnel might be useful in insuring that normal skills and capacities were not lost, or even in enhancing such skills or capacities. All such functions were "ancillary" to the "treatment" itself. But as soon as one sees, as did Stanton and Schwartz, that what goes on in the immediate hospital environment, whether the patient is aware of it or not is related to the waxing and waning of the symptoms for which he is being treated, the meaning of treatment changes sharply. The doctor is no longer in isolation with the patient; the total environment they share influences the process of what goes on between them and influences the course of the patient's movement.

Thus, the above studies show that there are environmental structures which can enhance, and that there are environmental structures which can discourage the process by which the psychologically alienated person makes his way back to "normal" society. Presumably then, environments can be created which ease, or at least, do not interfere with this process. The halfway house may be seen as one attempt to establish environments appropriate to certain stages of psychological need and certain stages of psychological development. Along with other innovations, the halfway house represents a search for more tenable alternatives to the hospital model.

Changing Conceptions of "Mental Illness"

The preceding pages have suggested that the notion of psychological disturbance as a disease comparable to other diseases is fallible. All who have had anything to do with the problem— whether as patient, as friend or relative of the victim, or as policeman, lawyer, judge, or witness in legal issues of insanity, or as professional working with the sufferer—have, fully aware or not, trembled and floundered on the shaky ground of this notion.

It would be specious to deny the historical and social importance of the disease concept to the mentally disturbed. At least in theory it is far better to be a patient than a pariah, an outcast, a maniac, a wild animal. And compared to being a hopeless case, at best locked in an attic, it is—again, at least in theory—hopeful and humane to be sick in a hospital. Nor would we hesitate to choose between eighteenth century bedlam and the modern psychiatric hospital, or between the goals of incarceration and those of cure.

Moreover, there is an inducement for the community in the "sickness" concept. When the community defines someone as ill, the physician takes over. There is comfort, sad comfort though it is, in the idea that the madman is ill. Illness removes at least a bit of the mystery of aberration and some of the personal horror. One calls for the doctor. Some mystery remains, as with diseases we know little about, and responsibility and misery are by no means dissipated. Still it is a comfort to know John's illness is not himself, and that his talk and actions are really not his but rather the products of a "sick" mind, and that no one is really at fault And there is always hope that a new and quick cure will be found.[6] Nevertheless, whatever the historical and social usefulness of the medical concept of mental illness, the question may be raised of how well it has worked in practice. And doubts may be expressed about the cost at which it has been purchased.

In simple, practical terms, because of the ambiguities noted above, there are persistent tendencies for the mental hospital to regress to its earlier forms. Periodic cries for hospital reforms—of Dorothea Dix in the 1880's, Clifford Beers in the 1920's, Albert Deutsch in the 1940's and 50's, all laymen we may note—have transient effects. Hospitals revert to the condition of prisons and worse. Even more important, however, is the question of the scientific price of the medical concept. For if we labor under inadequate or false concepts, we exact from sufferers of today and of

---

[6] It is a hard soul who would deny the sufferer and those who suffer with and for him these small comforts, though those dedicated workers who have chosen to vie with madness in tedious, demanding daily battle have had to be—if they were to help—such hard souls, choosing reality over comfort.

the future the hope of a changed condition. They and our works, however well-meaning, are squandered.

If the fundamental concepts and the assumptions they entail are bad, then hospital reform is no answer. Attempts to modify and augment programs for treating psychological disturbance, and at the same time maintain an orientation appropriate to sickness, are ingenious and at times heroic. But the result of such attempts is that legitimate notions of the importance of the social and physical milieu, and of ways to modify the environment so as to increase the likelihood of an improvement in thought and action, are degraded into prescriptions. Just as a drug is prescribed, so now we prescribe "*a* therapeutic milieu."

An example is patient self-government. One can defend self-government on simple, humanitarian grounds. People have a right—except under the most unusual circumstances—to participate in the decisions which affect them. Or one may speak of experiments in self-government as part of a training process whereby those who have had considerable difficulty in their associations with others are given opportunity for interpersonal explorations in a benign, supportive, and sometimes specially helpful context. Sivadon, for example, plans for his patients to engage in an orderly sequence of such explorations in accordance with a sophisticated notion of the course of development of object relations. What is not tenable is the mystique whereby self-government is seen as in ingredient of a new wonder drug called "therapeutic milieu."

Such confusions are apt to arise from the word "therapy" and its associations with sickness. As the Cummings note, in traditional medicine patients are passive recipients of help. Where the patient is ". . . actor, initiator, cooperator, and manager of his own affairs and [others are] assistants . . . (Cumming & Cumming, 1962, p. 138)," the notion of patient and doctor is apt to be confusing. And where democracy is seen as "healthy" from a medical rather than ethical or educational point of view, the muddle increases. Even in so sophisticated a setup as Maxwell Jones' there was considerable confusion as to the functions of self-government (Rapaport, 1960).

Self-government or therapeutic milieu are not prescriptions to be filled out by a staff and swallowed by a patient. What is helpful in an environment depends on what one needs and wants. A resort hotel, for example, is useful to many people, although no good hotel would undertake to be governed by its guests. The conceptual orientation toward a model of "sickness" pulls thoughtful and legitimate innovations into mindless clichés. And what is of value in recent notions of "therapeutic milieu" and "therapeutic community" is aborted because of the medical dilemma.

The dilemma is no less in individual therapy. At times it seems as though in those hospitals where individual treatment is emphasized, patients and doctors must have a secret pact with one another. While overtly going along with the rules of the medical game in their work with each other, they share the secret that the game is irrelevant and its rules absurd. The nurses and attendants who take the game seriously—and for whom primarily the game at times seems to be played—are tossed into an ambiguous and highly uncomfortable situation. Like the person tricked into a phony game where the overt rules are one thing and the covert rules another, they are caught in the middle. They escape their predicament by quitting or by denying their suspicions and pretending that nothing really is going on—a solution which predisposes either to apathetic withdrawal by staff or to total tyranny. Or they may gradually become privy to the secret, sharing in the collusion, so that they can come to play the real game effectively. The overt system and its selection devices make this latter solution all too rare. That some true helpers emerge is a tribute to virtue and integrity.

Although the dilemmas inherent in the medical conceptualization of "mental illness" had been noted before—often in informal conversation among professionals, seldom in formal presentations—it is a psychiatrist, Thomas Szasz, who in public forum faced these issues bravely, clearly, and cogently. Szasz (1961) suggests that the notion of mental illness makes historical but not rational sense, and that in a rational sense the notion is scientifically worthless and socially harmful. He points out that part of the usefulness of a class name is that it includes only a few things. Valuable distinctions are lost when all sorts of manifestations are labeled illness, just as they would be if we were to call all colors green. Szasz notes: "At first, [illness] was composed of only a few items, all of which shared the common feature of reference to a state of disordered structure or function of the human body as a physicochemical machine. As time went on, additional items were added to this class. They were not added, however, because they were newly discovered bodily disorders. The physician's attention had been deflected from this criterion and had become focused instead on disability and suffering as new criteria for selection. Thus, at first slowly, such things as hysteria, hypochondriasis, obsessive-compulsive neurosis, and depression were added to the category of illness. Then, with increasing zeal, physicians and especially psychiatrists began to call 'illness' . . . anything and everything in which they could detect any sign of malfunctioning, based on no matter what norm. Hence, agoraphobia is illness because one should not be afraid of open spaces. Homosexuality is illness because heterosexuality is the social norm. Divorce is illness because it signals the failure of marriage. Crime, art, undesired political leadership, participation in social affairs, or withdrawal from such participation—all these and many more have been said to be signs of mental illness (p. 44–45)."

Szasz comments on other discrepancies between legitimate criteria for physical and those for "mental illness." For example, in most illnesses, the sufferer defines himself as sick; in "mental illness" he is often so defined against his will. Furthermore, in "mental," but not in physical illness, emphasis is placed on economic, political and ethical considerations; as in the case of the witches in Salem, the criterion becomes antisocial behavior, growing out of, and relevant to, a particular social context. Szasz does not deny that bodily illnesses may be favored by certain social manifestations—tuberculosis being favored by poverty, for instance, or venereal diseases by promiscuity. But, he notes, once physical disease occurs, the symptoms are independent of social considerations. Presumably, too, the treatments for a particular ailment should be the same. Certainly this is not so for "mental illness." We mentioned previously Hollingshead and Redlich's (1958) telling analysis of divergencies in "treatment" based on social class differences. It would be absurd to believe that economic considerations do not affect the quality of treatment one is likely to receive for physical illness; but it is only with "mental disease" that they affect the very form and nature of "treatment."

Szasz argues that, rather than with diseases, psychiatry deals with problems of living; that one cannot, in this sense, talk of "treatment" and "cure"; that ". . . psychotherapy is an effective method of helping people—not to recover from an 'illness,' it is true, but rather to learn about themselves, others, and life (Preface, p. xi)." He suggests that the labeling of suffering as illness delayed recognition of the relevant phenomena and limited the kinds of questions which could be asked.

In his own conceptualization, Szasz has moved toward thinking of the categories of psychological disturbance as representing aberrant systems of communication. The problem of change (rather than "cure") is analogous to that of shifting from one language into another. Hysteria, for example, he suggests is a language learned and used like other language. Such concepts are similar to ones being developed by Bateson, Jackson, Haley, & Weakland (1956, 1963), Bowen (1960), Lidz, Fleck, & Cornelison (1965), and Wynne, Ryckoff, Day, & Hirsch (1958), Wynne and Singer (1963a, 1963b) for the more debilitating disturbances, such as schizophrenia. Each of these investigators suggest that fundamental to the phenomena of schizophrenia are histories of disruptive family communication patterns.

It is far too early, in terms of available evidence, to judge the validity of these newer conceptualizations. At present there exist no irrefutable conclusions on the etiology of schizophrenia (cf. Rosenthal, 1963; Jackson, 1960). Arguments have been made for genetic factors, but the studies supporting such factors have been questionable. Furthermore, studies which are well controlled have not succeeded in identifying biochemical, physiological or anatomical features as fundamental to schizophrenia. The effectiveness of drugs, or of physical methods, such as electro-shock therapy, constitutes no argument in favor of, or opposed to, any particular theory of causes. That drugs and physical trauma can have profound psychological effects is true for "normals" as well as for "schizophrenics." To argue from such effects toward a theory of physical etiology and physical treatment for psychological phenomena is but another instance of the mind-body and illness-health confusions which have hindered scientific advance.

The recent conceptualizations—such as Szasz's—of mental disturbance offer no unequivocal answers. But they have cleared the ground for another way of thinking and for another form of experimentation. Wittingly or unwittingly, innovations in dealing with living conditions and arrangements and with the social experiences of the disturbed are social experiments. Szasz points out that Pinel's liberation of patients at Salpêtrière was not an innovation in medical treatment, but rather a social reform. So, too, modifications in the environments of hospitals are social and not medical experiments. That they are grafted onto medical assumptions restricts and confounds the nature and the interpretation of these experiments. The halfway house, having moved a greater distance from the medical milieu, offers a new field for studying and for helping solve some of the problems of living for those who have suffered severe psychological upset.

Chapter 3   TOWARD A DEFINITION
OF THE HALFWAY HOUSE

In one sense there would seem to be little need to search for a definition of the halfway house. The term "halfway" defines itself. And the previously mentioned descriptions—Huseth's (1962), Reik's (1953), Wechsler's (1960)—are consistent with one another. Each suggests that the halfway house is a transitional living facility, intermediate between mental hospital and community. Furthermore, all three descriptions imply a single direction of movement. That is, the halfway house serves the ex-patient moving *from* the hospital *to* the community. The brochures of various facilities describing themselves as halfway houses show similar consistency. Although these most often give no formal definitions, there is a striking and recurrent use of the terms "bridge" and "transition." Suggestions by such authors as Wechsler (1960) of a continuum of "quarter-way," "half-way," and "three-quarter-way" houses contain similar implications.

By the word *definition* we shall mean more than this. Our search is toward a description based on actual operations. As Neff (1964) notes, it is only after we achieve the descriptive details of goals and operations that we can be in a position to evaluate effectiveness so as to draw rational and useful conclusions. Preliminary description requires knowing what halfway houses are like—what they do, how they do it, who they serve, and who does the serving.

There are two ways of achieving such descriptions, and both are necessary. One approach involves the micro-analysis of a particular institution. Through such an approach, description can come close to giving the intimate raw details of what actually goes on. The knowledgeable reader of such a description is in a position to check the author's inferences, to examine consistencies and inconsistencies, and to draw his own conclusions. If he can assume that the institution is representative, or if he has sufficient background to make legitimate comparisons, he can derive critical generalizations from a detailed intimate description.

Such descriptions are needed for halfway houses. As we have seen in the case of hospitals, vague statements of general goals and idealized versions of administrative procedures can mask the actualities of daily experience. And it is the masking of these actualities which obstructs further knowledge. Some of the operational details of halfway houses can be gleaned from reports and publications, and at least one book presenting an intimate description of the development of a halfway house and of its course of daily life has appeared (Rothwell & Doniger, 1966; see also Landy & Greenblatt, 1965). More such studies are needed.

A second form of description attempts to survey a broad field. What it cannot achieve in intimacy of detail, the survey study compensates for in breadth of scope. Where—as in the case of halfway houses—there is wide variability among institutions and detailed information is obscure, the survey is an efficient source of knowledge. It is limited by its reliance on what people say they do, rather than on observation of what they actually do. But if we can assume adequate questions, appropriate sampling, and capable and honest replies, the survey enables generalizations and comparisons which could not otherwise be easily achieved.

Most of the material which follows derives from a survey of halfway houses conducted in early and mid-1963. The respondents were directors and administrators of halfway houses. The inferences to be drawn thus come from "official" sources. Whether the residents themselves would paint similar pictures is, of course, an open question and one which needs investigation. Our aim here must be to provide only a broad map of the topography of halfway houses, and to infer what we can about the potentialities of the terrain. That such an exploration in no way substitutes for a detailed mapping of each section makes it no less essential.

We did, however, attempt to check our maps. Where appropriate, the interpretation of respondents' replies to questions about their halfway houses is supplemented by other sources of information. Among these sources are brochures and published or unpublished reports of specific halfway houses, and formal and informal discussion with halfway house workers over the country; a more active participation in a particular halfway house—Woodley House in Washington, D. C.—was particularly useful.

Defining the Sample

In order to conduct a survey, one must decide who is to be surveyed. Thus, even initially, there is a matter of definition. A survey of halfway houses requires some preliminary notions of what is and what is not a halfway house.

We have already noted the commonly mentioned "bridge" or "transition" component of definitions. But the descriptions in the literature referred to above usually imply some additional aspects which serve to differentiate halfway houses: (*a*) the residents have recognized psychiatric problems; (*b*) the halfway house is usually not on hospital grounds; (*c*) it is, if only temporarily, the primary residence of the persons living there; and (*d*) residents presumably do not stay permanently in a halfway house.

These rather vague criteria formed an initial base for selection of the population of halfway houses. Several other criteria, some of which are implicit above, entered into the selection. For the purpose of the study, all facilities defined as halfway houses maintain something of a professional orientation. This might vary from actual staffing of houses with members of one or more of the "mental health" professions to use of professionally trained personnel solely in an advisory or consultant capacity. The "professional" criterion thus eliminates the more informal types of boarding houses, and the study can yield no indication of their prevalence.

Furthermore, the selection is confined to houses whose purpose is in serving the needs of those with direct psychological problems. Eliminated from consideration are houses whose primary purpose is to serve the needs of alcoholics, or narcotic addicts, or released prisoners. Facilities for these latter populations have developed rapidly in the last several years (Blacker & Kantor, 1960; Breslin & Crosswhite, 1963), but the problems dealt with are sufficiently different to require separate study. For the same reason a few houses devoted to geriatric patients or to the mentally deficient were also eliminated.

The practical problem of obtaining lists of respondents who met in several ways. An initial working list was obtained from Woodley House, a halfway house in Washington, D. C., whose personnel had been in contact, through correspondence and visits, with personnel of other halfway houses.[1] The original list was supplemented by information obtained from directors of the halfway houses on the initial working list. The Central Offices of the Veterans Administration and of the Office of Vocational Rehabilitation were consulted for additional information, and further suggestions were elicited from the National Institute of Mental Health.[2] A final check of facilities was made at a conference on halfway houses held in Washington, D. C., in May of 1963.

The Sample

In this fashion a list of some 71 possible facilities was obtained. Not all of these were known to exist. For example, in some

[1] We are indebted to Edith Maeda and Joan Doniger for their help in this phase.

[2] We are indebted to Miss Ruth I. Knee of the Community Services Branch of NIMH.

cases questionnaires were mailed out on the basis solely of hearsay evidence that someone was thinking of starting a halfway house. Where more than one facility was administered by the same institution, each facility was initially considered as independent. Presumably, every halfway house in the country falling within the above criteria was approached.

Each of these possible facilities was sent a questionnaire (APPENDIX A). A face sheet described the purposes of the study and included a request for notification about other halfway houses in the area. A return envelope was enclosed. If no reply was received, a follow-up letter, accompanied by another copy of the questionnaire, was sent in about three weeks. If necessary, a second follow-up letter was mailed after three additional weeks.

In all, replies were received from 57 respondents. Of these, seven were not operating halfway houses at the time, although several were interested or involved in the process of beginning one. Nine houses did not meet the criteria, being halfway houses for drug addicts or alcoholics, or day-care centers for psychiatric patients. One house sent a brochure but did not complete the questionnaire.

Six institutions operated two halfway house facilities apiece. The final sample (APPENDIX B) thus represents 40 halfway houses under the direction of 34 managements. An informal check with halfway house directors well distributed over the country yielded a subjective estimate that only four houses which might possibly have met the criteria failed to reply.

The Questionnaire

The literature on halfway houses and an acquaintance with the operation of Woodley House furnished the basis for the design of the questionnaire. The earlier questionnaires used by Wechsler (1960) and by Ghan (1962) were a prime initial source for items.[3]

[3] Thanks are due Dr. Henry Wechsler of the Massachusetts Mental Health Center for furnishing this questionnaire.

For purposes of data analysis and comparability, objective items were favored wherever feasible. Such items were supplemented by requests for more open-ended information, and at the end of the questionnaire a section allowed for spontaneous comments. That the respondents took a serious interest in the study is suggested by the elaborate and detailed comments many of them chose to make.

In its final form the questionnaire covered nine major areas: (*a*) origins and population; (*b*) staff; (*c*) physical plant; (*d*) rules; (*e*) financial arrangements; (*f*) work and jobs; (*g*) therapy; (*h*) discharge; (*i*) community relations.[4] These sections of the questionnaire form much of the basis for the chapters which follow.

---

[4] Mrs. Naomi Rothwell was especially helpful in the design of the questionnaire.

Chapter 4   THE DEVELOPMENT
AND INITIATION OF
HALFWAY HOUSES

THE QUESTIONNAIRE ASKED RESPONDENTS FOR THE DATE OF ESTAB-
lishment of their halfway house, how and by whom it came to be
established, and at a later point, about community attitudes toward
the establishment of the halfway house.

The Growth of the Movement

We have already noted the progressively rapid development of halfway houses. The trend is clearly seen in the 40 houses
of the sample. Before 1954, and before the term "halfway house"
came into popular usage, there were only three such facilities—
Gould Farm in Massachusetts founded in 1913, Spring Lake Ranch
in Vermont founded in 1932, and Meadowlark Homestead in
Kansas founded in 1951. All three of these institutions were in rural
settings. All were founded through the individual inspiration of
concerned nonprofessionals. Although it is doubtful that their
founders were conscious of this, each of the facilities harked back to
that enlightened, early 19th century period of "moral treatment."
All were, in a sense, spiritual retreats. The orientation was less
psychiatric, or even psychological, than humanistic. A return to the

49

virtues of a simpler, more natural, more loving life was emphasized. Two of the institutions, Gould Farm and Meadowlark Homestead, emphasized and continue to emphasize religious motives. All stressed the spiritual benefits to be found in work and in cooperative living. All three facilities are active to this day.

The modern era of urban halfway houses may be said to have begun in 1954 with the conversion of Rutland Corner House from a temporary residence and rehabilitation center for homeless or indigent "decent" women to a psychologically oriented halfway house (Landy, 1960; Landy & Greenblatt, 1965; Lyman, 1961). Since then, the number of halfway houses has consistently accelerated. More than 60% of the forty houses in the sample were started after 1960. In 1962 alone, eight new houses, one-fifth of the sample, were founded and by early spring of 1963, when the present study was undertaken, there were already four additional houses.

How They Get Started

There are no specific items in the questionnaire which provide a full answer to the question of how halfway houses get started. Some information can, however, be gleaned from items dealing with the purpose of the house, financial aspects, and community relations, and from spontaneous comments.

The ways of initiation and the sources of encouragement and backing are many and diverse. As with the early rural houses, in a number of cases interested and highly motivated individuals sought out people and organizations who could supply professional and financial resources. Of the forty houses in the sample, nine seemed to have their origin in such specifically individual impetus. Some of these pioneers began entirely on their own—sometimes after failure to find organizational support—taking personal responsibility for the financing. An example is Woodley House, where the persistent determination of one person culminated in the founding of the first professionally oriented house in the Washington, D. C. area. A succinct description is given by Joan Doniger (Doniger, 1964).

> In the 1940's, on the first day of my first job as an occupational therapist in the mental hospital, my new colleagues and I told each other at lunch that, as far as we could see, many of the people in the hospital didn't need to be there. As the years passed I changed jobs, but the luncheon conversations didn't change. After about thirteen years of the same talk, the time came to do something. Also, by this time, there were four or five halfway houses in existence . . . It wasn't a particularly new idea; many writers had already shown that social structures of hospitals were not necessarily ideal for the care of the mentally ill—and the halfway house fitted the trend toward community psychiatry. In 1958 a few ex-colleagues from NIH and I formed the non-profit corporation . . . which then established Woodley House with $3000 of borrowed money.

The houses which started earlier often owed their inception to intensive individual efforts. But most houses, particularly the later ones, were begun by organizations which sought out individuals to carry through and staff a project conceptualized by the organization's leaders. There is considerable variety among organizations taking the initiating steps. Five of the halfway houses of the sample evolved from the efforts of local mental health associations or rehabilitation organizations; six began with the backing of state vocational rehabilitation offices; two others were begun under county or state auspices; four houses were started through the action of local charitable organizations or foundations; in the largest single category, fourteen houses originated with the Veterans Administration. Since the halfway house represents a borderland area between professional psychiatric care facilities and the social community, very often more than a single organization is involved. An example is the cooperation between the Vermont State Hospital and the State Vocational Rehabilitation Division in establishing halfway houses at Montpelier and Burlington.

Whatever the source of initiation, once the house exists, other sources of support are very often drawn in. In early stages private donations and foundation support may play an important role. A major source of beginning support for some houses has been demonstration grants from the National Vocational Rehabilitation Administration and from NIMH, although these administrations did not themselves initiate the halfway house.

Initial Relations with the Community

Where a need for transitional facilities exists and where individuals and organizations are willing to meet this need, it might seem that communities would be accepting in their attitudes and eager to have halfway houses added to their resources. Such a view is, of course, naive. People may favor the idea of a halfway house, but, like a fire department, no one wants it next door.

Of the forty houses represented in the survey, seventeen report some kind of trouble in relation to the community at the beginning of the project. The extent of difficulties varied. They ranged from inquiries which required only friendly and reassuring answers from the halfway house staff, to the swearing out by an organized neighborhood committee of a court order to have the halfway house removed. Two houses, neither of which are included in the sample of forty, had been forced to close. In both, the residents had engaged in behavior intolerable to the community. One house had accepted overt homosexuals; at the other house one of the residents committed a rape and murder.

Even under less dramatic circumstances, the halfway house is apt to face impediments in its initial relations with the community. The obstructions may be so massive as to force a change of plans, and we do not know how many potential halfway houses are lost at this initial stage. Sometimes community opposition compels a change of plans for the location of the halfway house. A case in point comes from Kentucky (Meenach, 1964):

> At one site we selected, the climate of the neighborhood was unfriendly. Efforts . . . to prove to the neighborhood that this was a worthwhile project that would not alter anyone's everyday living in

the neighborhood failed. . . . We found the greatest objection was not the purpose of the project but fear, devaluation of property, encroachment on a residential area. . . . We found that the general attitude of each city was favorable and offered moral support through organizations and letters to the editors of local papers and contact with the members of the Advisory Board. But this did not mean establishment was smooth sailing. When the fact was known that a halfway house would be established, opposition was immediately put into action (pp. 13–14).

The description goes on to speak of petitions by residents of the neighborhood culminating in a change of site.

Not all halfway houses undergo such intense initial contests. A successfully resolved difficulty of the Vermont Rehabilitation Unit in Montpelier (Brooks, 1959; Chittick, Brooks, Irons,& Deane, 1961) is worth summarizing: The Rehabilitation Division of the State of Vermont, in cooperation with the Vermont State Hospital, was engaged in the preparation of a Rehabilitation House, when knowledge of this new development spread to the surrounding community, and resistance began to be organized. The neighbors feared violence; they feared that children would not be safe in the area; and they feared that their property values would go down. When this uproar threatened, the Rehabilitation Division and the Hospital both enlisted the aid of the newspapers and the local clergy to lead in discussion of what the house was trying to accomplish and what it really meant for the community. Very shortly, opposition died down and more understanding attitudes took its place.

A similar experience is reported in St. Louis (Kohler, Bandle, Ossorio, Schumacher, 1962):

The first sign of community resistance was stimulated by a local organization composed primarily of landlords in the immediate neighborhood. This group sent inquiries to the Department of Safety of the St. Louis City Hall. The Mental Hygiene Association then received a letter inquiring as to the nature of the house and indicating the resistance of this organization to having mental patients living in the community. This was solved by the MHA members who contacted leaders of this organization, as well as the City Hall representative, and invited them for lunch and a tour of the halfway house. There was enthusiastic response and this group never posed a danger to establishing a house in the community (p. 5).

How to Approach the Community

In initiating relations with the community, administrators have used varying approaches, ranging from a conscious effort to avoid initial contact to an active seeking of contact. Some houses have announced their specific purposes before opening. Others have never discussed it at all with the surrounding community even after the house has been operating for several years—avoiding publicity out of the wish to preserve to as great an extent as possible the anonymity of the house.

Where the choice is toward an open public statement, there are a number of possible tactics. Some of these are suggested above in the illustrations of reactions to community opposition. But if one is going to tackle the problem openly, it is probably better to do so before overt opposition organizes:

> The Gutman House in Portland, Oregon, a week before its opening, extended invitations to an Open House, in person to all neighbors within a two-block radius. They gave the neighbors a one-page fact sheet describing the nature and purpose of the house. Twenty percent of those invited attended the Open House. A tour was given, refreshments were served, and all questions were answered. There has been no opposition to the House expressed by the community in its first three months of operation (Gutman House Progress Report, 1963, p. 3).

Meenach (1964) suggests even more elaborate pre-planning:

> . . . we recommend that the city officials, newspapers, members of the neighborhood, church groups, clubs, and key individuals be fully informed and understand the purpose and function of the

project. An important asset is to involve the community as much as possible. Form an advisory committee of key citizens very early in your developing stages. Your early advisory group can later appoint key members in addition to the earlier group. We found that the community resented a public agency forcing itself into the community like a highway. Therefore, if the project can evolve from the community itself, this is ideal . . . Keep your information simple, and truthful. Make an effort to enlighten, inform, and instruct the community (p. 16).

As noted, other houses have preferred to avoid and have succeeded in avoiding a public focus. Woodley House presents an example (Doniger, 1964):

There was a lot of discussion about how to prepare the neighborhood for our arrival. We heard that other halfway houses had difficulties and were warned that it would be wise to allay the neighbor's fears about us. We didn't do it. We moved in quietly. Many of our neighbors still don't know who we are or what we are doing. The trouble with asking too many people's permission is that you may not get it. Publicity gives people a chance to mobilize their defenses; it doesn't matter what you want to do, there's always somebody against it. Well-known public agencies, of course, don't often have the freedom to operate as quietly as we did. Also, we probably would not have been as inconspicuous in a small town or homogeneous residential neighborhood and might therefore have had a greater initial public relations job to do. We did have to tell our prospective landlord the use we intended to make of his property. When he learned that, he did not want to lease the house to us and it took considerable time and effort to convince him to do so. He has found us [to be] satisfactory tenants.

There is obviously no clear agreement among halfway houses about initial attitudes and procedures in relation to the community. Certainly studies are needed for determining the efficacy of alternative modes of approach. Nonetheless, the choice is not entirely an arbitrary one. As Doniger hints, a major determinant is the structure and character of the neighborhood. At one extreme are the rural houses. If these are self-sufficient in operations, if residents engage in no contact with the environs, there may be little need for a campaign for community support and approval. If, on the other hand, the facility seeks opportunities for employment, recreation, and social relations for its residents in the neighboring community, the focalization of the community must be not merely toward tolerance but toward active involvement. In a small town, or in a well-established, stable residential community in a large city, the halfway house cannot avoid public confrontation. It is advisable that the confrontation be planned for and that leaders of the local community become allies for the inevitable conflict to come. Quite different, however, are highly urbanized, somewhat transitional neighborhoods in large cities. An example is that of Woodley House: ". . . a busy, mind-your-own-business one in which apartments, hotels, boarding houses, stores, and private homes are mixed . . . in a middle-class section of the city." Another example are the apartments maintained by Fountain House in New York City (Beard, Schmidt, Smith, & Dincin, 1964). Such houses do not depend on the immediate local neighborhood for work or social opportunities. Because such neighborhoods are anonymous, the house can more easily maintain its own anonymity.

For most of the sample the majority of difficulties in relation to the community have been resolved through time and/or continuous interpretation. Many house directors, however, continue to feel that some incident might easily activate problems with the community, bringing about an active and hostile concern. It is well to recognize that community fears are not wholly illegitimate. As *Action for Mental Health* (1961) notes, the unattractive behavior of the psychologically disturbed is a barrier to community sympathy.

Attitudes of the Professional Community

In contrast to local neighborhoods, one might expect strong positive support from the professional community. Where the house is integrated from the start with a mental hospital or with community clinics, there is such support. For the individually established halfway house it is not always immediately forthcoming. Wayne (1963) reports:

> First, how receptive is the psychiatric profession to rehabilitation programs? In our initial months the most encompassing problem was massive apathy in the professional community. While we received many accolades from the profession for our pioneering effort in rehabilitation, few psychiatrists made use of the facility. For months we functioned at only a fraction of capacity. Psychiatrists were often unable to identify patients who might benefit from a halfway house.
>
> In other instances, to put it bluntly, psychiatrists were apprehensive about using the halfway house. Even though residents at Edgemont House are not required to be in treatment with staff therapists . . . , many of our colleagues seemed to suspect that their relationships with their patients might be interrupted, or diluted, or in some way tampered with.
>
> To overcome these difficulties, we undertook an educational program directed to the mental health professions. We took our story to meetings of professional groups, prepared descriptive literature, invited therapists to visit us and observe our program in action. Barriers are now breaking down. Referrals are building, not only from psychiatrists in the community but from others with treatment responsibility (p. 441).

Woodley House reports similar experiences. Token verbal support of professionals was not lacking. But only after a number of newspaper stories and public talk did active professional involvement ensue.

In summary, then, halfway houses begin with sometimes heroic efforts of an individual or an organization. Initial financial support is often tenuous, and communities are not likely to be receptive. If the halfway house is to be located in a stable residential neighborhood, considerable preparation of the community is called for; if the neighborhood is highly urbanized, mixed residential and business, and transitional, it may be simpler for the halfway house to preserve anonymity. Even the professional mental health community may offer minimal real support unless special efforts are made to educate professionals. In spite of these difficulties the number of halfway houses has accelerated rapidly since 1954, and the acceleration seems to continue.

Part

II

STRUCTURES

A GOOD PART OF THE DISCUSSION IN CHAPTER 2 CONSIDERED SOME structural features of the mental hospital, and examined the impact of hospital structure on the mental sufferer. We noted, for example, that, as the physical and social distance between the mental hospital and the community increased, the functions of the hospital—along with its staff and inmates—decayed. We also saw how the internal structure of hospitals, with its emphasis on wards and beds, influenced attitudes and actions. So, too, hospital administrative structure and its particular gradations were seen to pattern and limit communication.

The present is a time of rapid reform and modification. Hospitals are changing and further changes are in the offing. In recent years the Joint Commission on Mental Illness and Health has proposed some major shifts of direction (*Action for Mental Health*, 1961). The Commission recognizes that the large mental hospital is outmoded. It suggests that new hospitals have no more than a thousand beds. It proposes that hospitals be integrated into the community as intensive treatment centers. It recognizes the debilitating effects of long-term institutionalization. It encourages efforts to avoid these effects and to return the patient to the community as soon as possible. It recommends flexible and intensive

programs of aftercare for the ex-patient. Evolving from the outlines of the Joint Commission's findings are comprehensive community mental health centers with panoramic networks of service.
Such transformations cannot but be welcomed.

Unfortunately, many of the current changes—salutary
though they may be—are superimposed on an old structural model.
All too few are structural innovations. In Chapter 2 we saw how
factors in the hospital-medical structure enhanced certain functions
and inhibited others. And sociological research implies that, in spite
of the best intentions, outmoded structures will continue to pervert
consciously desired goals.

The hospital structure and its hierarchies are realities
which, as Rothwell and Doniger (1963) suggest, must limit reforms. Token gestures of informality, experimental blurring of
roles, devices for patient government cannot, they indicate, oblit-
erate real distinctions. Within the hospital, the medical direction
and responsibility of the physician, the low paycheck of the attendant, the patient as seeker of care—all of these are indisputable fact.
So long as clinics are clinics and hospitals are hospitals, goodwill,
noble intentions, and even adequate funding are not enough.

So, too, what a halfway house does and how it does it is
determined not only by its general aims but also by the opportunities and limits provided in its structure. The next several
chapters consider some of the structural aspects of halfway houses
in relation to what halfway houses aim to do and to what they
actually do. We begin here with ecological and physical factors and
then go to financial, demographic, and administrative aspects.

Chapter 5 STRUCTURAL ASPECTS
OF THE HALFWAY HOUSE:
ECOLOGICAL AND PHYSICAL
FEATURES

The Location of Halfway Houses

CURRENT ATTITUDES IN SOCIAL PSYCHIATRY—AND EVEN MORE IM-
portant, problems of securing adequate professional staff—insure
that mental hospitals will no longer be so entirely isolated from
the general community. New hospitals will probably be part of
integrated mental health units with multiple facilities for serving
the non-hospitalized as well as the hospitalized. These facilities
will, it is likely, be close to major urban centers, or alternatively,
convenient to a network of small communities. In considering
location, planners will no doubt also emphasize the need for opportunities for continuing education and research, and so favor university and urban settings. Greater use will be made of general
hospitals which already exist in the community, but whose services
need to be supplemented. At present there is nothing, other than
possible political considerations, likely to counter these trends.

But even under the most favorable circumstances there will
be a great lag in time before mental hospitals shift to become a
physical part of our urbanized centers. This is not true in the case
of halfway houses.

As may be seen in Table 1, by far the greatest proportion

of halfway houses are found in urban-residential areas. If we consider urban-commercial and urban-residential areas together, these categories include 80% of all the houses. The degree of urbanization reveals sharply the difference from the traditional location of mental hospitals. It reflects the increasing urbanization of the general population, but also suggests the transitional function halfway houses ascribe to themselves.

TABLE I.   Area Location of Halfway Houses

	N
On Hospital Grounds	1[a]
Urban Commercial	7
Urban Residential	25
Suburban	2
Rural	5
	40

[a] One house was included although it was on hospital grounds. The house was founded in 1956 and has been included in previous surveys. It is clearly a halfway house according to both its own conception and other criteria.

Urban sites facilitate relations with the community. Occupational and recreational opportunities are near at hand. Public transportation—often a difficulty in relation to hospitals—is generally available, giving residents, who are unlikely to have cars at their disposal, a simple way to get where they wish to go. The physical problems of entry into ordinary nonpatient life—working, meeting friends, shopping—are eased. On the basis of their experience the directors of two halfway houses in Kentucky offer suggestions as to location (Meenach, 1964). They recommend neighborhoods: (a) zoned for business, in or near a residential area; (b) within walking distance of shops, churches, etc.; (c) near city bus transportation; (d) having well-lighted streets, police patrols, etc.; (e) near food markets.

As noted by some halfway house administrators, a central urban location has yet another advantage. It confers a kind of anonymity on its residents, providing a sometimes useful relief from pressures for particular modes of participation. The resident, especially one recently discharged after an extended stay in a hospital, often needs a moratorium period in which he can explore his way. Because it offers choices among multiple possibilities of association, but makes no absolute demands for participation, the urban setting confers a kind of protection from too many social pressures.[1] One can move in or out of groups or from periphery to center and vice versa without too much to-do.

As suggested earlier, the central urban location may also protect the house from too much community focus. The "busy, mind-your-own business [neighborhood] in which apartments, hotels, boarding houses, stores and private homes are mixed (Doniger, 1964)" is less apt to feel threatened by the halfway house.

The five rural houses, which make up one-eighth of the sample, usually have larger grounds, more buildings and more residents. They tend to be self-sufficient in terms of both work and play. Consequently they are able to provide the resident with the option of either staying within the microcosmic world of the house or of attempting a transition between the house and the wider community. The scales may be weighted in favor of the former because of transportation problems and because of possibly greater resistance to strangeness in the small-town community. The self-sufficiency of the rural houses is likely, however, to enable them to accept a greater degree of psychological disturbance in residents than urban houses could. And to those residents they offer a simpler, less fragmented pattern of life than is possible in an urban setting. They thus may be able to serve some who could not get along in the complexities of city life with its varied stimuli and many choices.

In practice the rural houses tend to provide something

[1] Barker (1963) describes how small towns and small institutions pull greater participation from members than do their larger equivalents.

more. That is, if we oversimplify, we can say that the urban houses offer their residents opportunities for connecting with the common life of the community and they offer the support required for meeting these opportunities. Such a stand reveals no very special philosophical orientation—just an everyday pragmatic approach, though perhaps a more humanistic one than usual. On the other hand, there is a tendency for the rural houses to offer—although they do not demand—a way of life. In this they embody some of the qualities of the experimental utopias prevalent in the America of an earlier era. We have more to say of this later. Here we would note only the ecological consideration: that only in the self-sufficient rural setting is the communal philosophy likely to be fostered and maintained.

Architectural Aspects

Consider first the mental hospital. The following quote from a paper sponsored by the World Health Organization presents a picture which, though changing, is thoroughly familiar today.

The buildings, usually massive and only comparable with prisons or barracks, most commonly the former, are usually hideous. The size of the hospital dwarfs the surrounding houses. . . . It is common for the hospital to be approached by a stately drive which culminates in a direct approach to the centre of an enormous block of buildings. . . . Such buildings make the visitor feel small, powerless, and insignificant. The effect on the patient is to increase any tendency he may have to run away, to destroy this frightening object or such parts of it as he can, or to retreat into inert submission.

Once inside the door of the hospital the patient is usually taken from an entrance hall to a records department where his documents will be examined . . . After this he will be escorted down long corridors where he will see numbers of patients sitting or walking aimlessly, perhaps exhibiting gross evidence of desocialization and eccentricity. He may then arrive at an admission unit where he will be examined by a doctor before being taken to yet another unit which will be his ward for initial observation and treatment. He will be put to bed and left to observe his surroundings. . . . In nearly all existing hospitals the wards are identical and arranged in a strongly formal way along a series of corridors either parallel to or radiating from a centre. This means that there is very little easy identification of place by the mental patient. Once he leaves his ward and starts wandering up and down the corridor there is nothing in the shape or design of the building to enable him to identify his own ward as against any other. . . . Many features of the design of older mental hospitals are continuous reminders to the patients that they are in custody. Apart altogether from such details as special locks on doors, bars on windows, windows designed to open only to a tiny extent, . . . quite a number of mental hospitals have very small windows, reminiscent of prisons, and many are also built of special materials or include special features in the design which remind patients that they are in custody and are expected to smash things and behave in a dirty or violent manner (Baker, Davies, & Sivadon, 1959, pp. 44–46).

The architecture of halfway houses contrasts sharply with the above picture. Part of the contrast is that—unlike the hospital with its particular structural requirements of wards—for halfway houses there are no fixed architectural formats. Table 2 suggests the high degree of diversity possible for potential halfway house facilities:

TABLE 2.   Types of Structures Used for
Halfway Houses

	N
Town houses	4
Big old place	20
Big new place	3
Ex-hospital or convalescent home	3
Ex-hotel or motel	4
Ex-apartment house	I
Rural farm buildings	3
On hospital grounds	I
Apartments	I
	40

Half of the forty houses are big old residences of the kind built originally to house the larger family groupings customary in the earlier decades of this century. The size of these houses enables them to accommodate sometimes as many as twenty residents. But at the same time their homelike architectural qualities make them particularly suitable for halfway house use. Such houses are often readily available in urban-residential areas, and their cost is likely to be considerably less than that of new construction of similar size.

Other houses have capitalized creatively on some unusual opportunities. For example, four houses utilize buildings which were previously hotels or motels. An unusual arrangement is that of Fountain House (Beard, Pitt, Fisher, & Goertzel, 1963) in New York. As part of a very diverse and extensive rehabilitation program, Fountain House maintains apartments scattered throughout New York City. The residents live in the apartments—two or three sharing an apartment—although they participate in other Fountain House activities at a single central location. The structural arrangements are thus characteristic of the highly urban New York community.[2] Still other houses use buildings which were formerly convalescent homes or small hospitals.

In furnishings, as in architecture, the halfway house contrasts greatly with the hospital. To quote again from the WHO description of hospitals:

> He [the patient] will see the many beds, all alike, and the absence of other furnishings, the walls of a dull, uniform institution buff or brown, and the windows small, high, barred and often dirty. . . . The ward will have a stale smell and often provide evidence of the inadequacy of the sanitary arrangements. He will also find within the ward no privacy, or opportunity to create it. He will be forced to perform even the most private activities where he can be seen by other patients and the staff. Within a crowd of such patients there

[2] By 1965, the number of apartments had grown to 22, almost doubling in two years. In addition, the Fountain House apartment arrangements now enable its program to serve mothers with small children (*Fountain House Progress Report*, 1965).

will be no opportunity to form friendships with a small group, or to feel any drive to identify himself with those around him. . . . The patients' quarters usually consist of large lofty rooms designed as open wards, together with tiny cells intended for seclusion, with no rooms of normal domestic proportions suitable for small family groups of people to sit together or eat together in a homely manner. . . . Indeed the accommodation for patients in existing mental hospitals is often deliberately designed to prevent the formation of small groups and to ensure that all patients are at all times under the eye of the nurse. Most of the patients' quarters in mental hospitals are designed on the assumption that there would be no furniture or only a very minimum of furniture. It is difficult today, now that it is recognized that patients should have cupboard accommodation for some of their possessions and clothes, to fit furniture into existing wards (Baker, Davies, & Sivadon, 1959, p. 45).

Certainly some parts of the above description would not fit many modern mental hospitals. But too much is true for even the best and newest hospital.

That halfway houses are much like homes is reflected in the great variability among them in room arrangements, furnishings, etc. Rooms may be large or small, many or few; furnishings may be modern, period or more usually nondescript; equipment may be old or new. But as with family homes there are some common features. For example, only six houses use dormitories at all. And only one of these has a dormitory with as many as five beds. As in usual middle-class adult society, people are generally in single or double rooms. The atmosphere is likely to be an open one. Few houses have rooms, other than the house-parent's or resident-manager's private one, which are kept closed, and in many houses even these are open. In a few cases some other rooms are closed to residents, usually because they store considerable amounts of household supplies or drugs. The free entry to the kitchen and use of kitchen equipment, books, and games, contrasts again with the hospital where everything must be asked for and where the normal facilities and freedom of a home are unavailable. In these respects the halfway house is very far from the hospital. On the other hand it is not quite a family home, although it may come close to seeming one. Architecturally its borders most often seem rather to lie in a nebulous region between family home and boarding house.

As closed, self-contained institutions, hospitals must provide all of the recreational facilities they deem necessary. Rural, farm-type halfway houses have a similar problem. Since these houses are the ones likely to have larger populations of residents, they can aim toward some degree of self-sufficiency in recreation. Urban halfway houses generally have no such aims. Here again they resemble a well-equipped home. Radio, television, newspapers are available, most often ping-pong, cards and games, and sometimes badminton or croquet courts and equipment if there is sufficient lawn space. As in a home, individual tastes enter. Often there is a piano, but one house had a harpsichord for a period of time.

The limitations in recreational facilities result not entirely from restrictions of space and finances: they are intended. The pursuit of other amusements—swimming, bowling, concerts, lectures, movies, plays, dances, tennis, spectator sports, and even beer-drinking at the nearest pub—all involve the resident with the community in interactions which may help him to resume life as a normal community member.

In the questionnaire some questions to respondents dealt with the degree of satisfaction they felt about their housing arrangements. Three categories for checking were available, followed by some open-ended questions. Twenty-seven of the forty houses report being very satisfied; the others report being somewhat satisfied; none find their arrangements unsatisfactory. The questions are indeed crude. Moreover, it should again be recognized that the questionnaire did not obtain the residents' viewpoints on these issues. Nonetheless it is interesting to note respondents' comments. Among the wished-for improvements are such things as: more space, more bathrooms, freer access to bathrooms, kitchen improvements, and better fireproofing. With the exception of the last item the list sounds very much like the average middle-class family householder's mild complaints. Like this householder the respondents express the optimistic belief that most of these improvements can be made in time. In any important sense, housing and architectural arrangements do not seem to offer critical problems for the administrators of halfway houses. We know of no comparable data, but we would guess that the same would not hold true for the administrators of mental hospitals.

We have devoted much attention here to architectural and ecological considerations. The topic is all too often neglected or skimmed over as one too superficial to merit close psychological scrutiny. Yet as we suggested in Chapter 2, a growing body of experience and study attests to its salience. The evidence is strong that hospitals inadvertently encourage the manifestations they aim to cure, and that contributing to this is the physical structure and ecology of the hospital. The authors of the WHO paper are not alone in feeling that: "Within this environment our patient feels no encouragement to develop human relationships, and he will see that his life is without purpose . . . regressive behavior will be reinforced by the architecture and by the regime which the design of the building tends to perpetuate (Baker, Davies, & Sivadon, 1959, p. 45)."

That the physical environment and its ecology make a difference in how people will think, act, and feel is confirmed by recent studies in human ecology (Barker, 1965), by studies of special conditions ranging from sensory isolation to concentration camp existence (Heron, 1957; Bettelheim, 1960), by suggestions from studies of animal ecology (Washburn & DeVore, 1961).

We can believe, but we cannot conclude that the halfway house offers something better in its architectural arrangements than does the hospital. To draw such a conclusion it would first be necessary to define what is meant by better, and then to proceed with empirical investigation. But we can say that the halfway house offers something different—something that comes closer to the model of family and home than does the hospital, and something predisposed to make a *resident* rather than a *patient*. We can point to the diversity among halfway houses and note that in such diversity there lies potential for study. For example, it is likely that certain houses, because of their location, their architecture, their furniture, will be more appropriate for certain types of residents than for others. Houses reflect social class, age, interests and values, and these may be fitting or unfitting, helpful or detrimental to the transition of particular residents. With increased knowledge one could hopefully plan specifically suitable environments for different segments of the population of the severely disturbed.

It would be a mistake to think of these issues as solely practical ones, for they have their basis in conceptual and theoretical considerations. It is out of a concept of mental disease that mental hospitals evolve, and the architecture and furnishings of such hospitals are derived from this concept. Family homes, too, are based on cultural concepts of what families represent—what and where are rights to privacy, what are the loci of interaction, what are the privileges associated with age, sex, or status—and homes in turn reflect these concepts. If our concepts of mental disturbance are changing, then our architecture is an anachronism. Conversely, if our architecture for the disturbed is deemed as needing change, it must be that our concepts are outdated. Winston Churchill once put the matter very succinctly: "We shape our buildings and later they shape us (quoted in Kling, 1959)."

Chapter 6   LEGAL AND FINANCIAL
STRUCTURE

Legal Structure

UNLIKE HOSPITALS OR NURSING HOMES, HALFWAY HOUSES HAVE
no tradition of legal precedents. For one thing, halfway houses are
yet too new, and as in other areas marked by significant recent
innovation, the laws governing their operation are unclear. Furthermore, as will be seen, there are no tight standards or restrictions
which define precisely what a halfway house should be. Both the hy-
brid character of halfway houses and the short duration of their operating existence mean that for the present, and very likely for some
time in the future, questions of legal status will remain ambiguous.

The legal ambiguity has some great present advantages.
It allows a degree of exploration which would otherwise be impossible. If standards of building, zoning, staffing, selection, and
responsibility were fixed, the variety among forms of halfway
houses would no doubt be sharply reduced. Since the diversity
represents and allows a search for better ways of living and for
more efficacious modes of integration with the community, curtail-
ment of variety would cut off opportunities for the disturbed. Even
more important, it would cut off sources for future practical and
theoretical knowledge.

Despite its advantages—which we believe essential to
maintain in at least the near future—legal ambiguity at times poses

some troublesome questions. Zoning, licensing, incorporation may present problems which are difficult to solve. Such matters must often be dealt with on a catch-as-catch-can basis suited to the local situation. Another area of ambiguity lies in the question of legal responsibility. Even for hospitals this question is a perplexing one, but for halfway houses the issues are even more confused. If residents are considered as patients on leave from their former hospitals, then the hospital has the legal responsibility for them. However, many residents do not have such leave status, and indeed many do *not* come directly from a mental hospital. Some houses require the resident's relatives to sign forms relieving the house of responsibility; the great degree of freedom permitted to residents in a halfway house system is thought to justify this procedure. Other houses reject such devices as too reminiscent of the medical-patienthood orientation. Even where waivers are signed there is doubt of their holding up in court; court cases would be subject to the vagaries of individual decisions. If, for example, a halfway house were found responsible for the illegal actions of a resident, the extent of penalty against the house might well depend upon whether the house was run for profit or whether it was—like most halfway houses—a nonprofit organization; profit-making institutions more commonly elicit severe judgment.

We know of no legal cases involving the professional responsibilities of halfway houses, and there is, perhaps fortunately, no background of legal experience for determining their status. How often would-be founders of halfway houses have been discouraged by these uncertainties is unknown. Administrators of halfway houses believe, however, that the legal risks are not sufficient to deter people who are really interested in establishing houses. Moreover, if legal issues were too worrisome, we would find houses selecting only well-behaved, low-risk residents. But though houses do set limits on whom they will take and on the degree of antisocial behavior they can tolerate, the limits are surprisingly broad. Within these limits there is—among those houses we know best—little or no effort to minimize risk; rather, there is a suggestion of pride in taking the more serious, the riskier, the more disruptive cases.

The indeterminate legal status does not seem to have distorted the professional goals of those who run halfway houses, though directors are nevertheless realistically cognizant of the twilight zone of legality in which they must operate. Houses often carry heavy and expensive insurance to provide for as many eventualities as possible. Since to operate within the limits of existing laws, strictly interpreted, would, in effect, violate the essential nature of the halfway house and transform it into a hospital, directors must come to terms with ambiguity. Since there are easier ways to make money than by running a halfway house, the situation no doubt selects only those who are strongly enough motivated to tolerate the absence of traditional supports and to make their own stands.

Financial Structure

Some comments about initial funding are in Chapter 4 in reviewing how halfway houses get started. Just as the auspices under which different houses were established were highly varied, so have been the sources of funds. Table 3 presents a categorization of initial approaches to financing. It is apparent that most houses (60%) were initiated with mostly personal financial resources. Such initial funds do not necessarily come from one individual; they include money borrowed from friends, and from financial

TABLE 3. Initial Primary Funding of Halfway Houses

	N
Personal	24
Federal Grants	9
State and County	4
Local Charitable Organizations	2
Veterans Administration	1
	40

organizations, and contributions from various sources. Nine of the forty houses—the next largest single category—were initiated as community demonstration and research projects with the aid of Federal grants.

These data deal with the primary source of initial funding. As such they indicate that, if present trends can be assumed to continue, the primary initial responsibility for fund raising will most often have to be personal, something anyone planning to start a halfway house needs to know. Moreover, experience suggests that this task is often difficult and demanding of time, energy and tact.

The figures can, however, be misleading. It is important to note that they represent only the principal source and only the starting point of funding. In a number of cases several sources of support made supplementary funds available. For 14 of the 24 houses which were begun with personal means, the Veterans Administration provided substantial support through referrals by the time the houses opened or very shortly thereafter.

Other houses have received Federal grant support at some later point in their development. In general, over the past decade houses providing professional services have had considerable support from branches of government and from benevolent foundations. Although aid is sometimes given at the inception of a project, more often it has come after the establishment of the house. A sizeable share of support has been given by the Federal government to demonstrate the demand for the services of halfway houses and to test their effectiveness in operation. When these studies are completed, however, houses may again find themselves operating at a deficit.

Except for one house, which was still a part of a VA hospital scheme, all houses in the survey charge fees. In about half the houses (21) there is a fixed schedule of fees; in the remaining houses (18) fees are based on ability to pay. At the houses with fixed fees, charges range from as low as $35 a month to as high as $700 ($700 for the first two months, $500 thereafter); the median fee is about $90 a month. Where fees are based on ability to pay, many residents pay nothing, and some pay as much as $650 a month; the house at the median has a range of fees between $0 and $140; the median fee for all such houses is slightly over $90 a month.[1]

Whether the fee schedule is fixed or variable, it presents a problem. Fixed fees exclude many from the opportunities of half-way house residence; they eliminate particularly those who are at present incapable of remunerative work and who lack families capable of contributing to their support. Winnowed out by fixed fees are the especially disabled and especially poor, a discrimination which goes counter to the social service orientation of many half-way house workers. But a fee structure based on the ability to pay presents another problem. The dilemma here is that the resident who goes out and gets a job and earns money will find himself paying higher fees as a result of his efforts. The situation is one familiar in welfare work, where the financial reward from gainful employment can be negated for the client by the equities established by the welfare system.

One attempt to solve the dilemma of variable fees is a kind of inverse fee system (Doniger, Rothwell, & Cohen, 1963). At Woodley House the more a resident works outside the house, the less rent he pays. Work is, however, not defined as necessarily remunerative. Paid work counts, but a volunteer job or going to school or even day-hospital attendance also counts as work. Any formal contribution of time which benefits resident or community is thus rewarded by lower rent. Woodley House finds that this approach does generally function as an incentive. When residents complain that they are penalized for being "sick," the answer is simply, "That's true." Moreover, the staff feels that there is a kind of fairness in the system. People who are around the house all day require more staff attention than do those who go to work.

In general, one detects among halfway house workers a sense of discomfort about fees. The discomfort is minimal when fees are paid by outside sources such as the Veterans Administration, but it rises when fees must be individually collected from each resident. Woodley House, for example, in response to staff tension

[1] It is important to note that these data are as of 1963.

about fees, finally turned over the setting and collecting of fees to a person not involved in the operation of the house. Such attempts at differentiation of roles may be useful in individual situations. They do not, however, resolve the fundamental problem of fees. A system which is seemingly based on ability to pay but which in practice operates to penalize efforts at productive work is inconsistent with the goals of halfway houses. On the other hand, an inverse fee schedule, such as at Woodley House, can have unfortunate consequences. It can function as a selection device by convertly favoring social adjustment and employability as criteria for admission to the house, eliminating the more severely disturbed. Moreover, it can be misused, as, for example, in the case of a resident who punished her parents, who were paying the fees, by insisting on working just short of the number of hours which would have reduced the fees. Still, the effort to relate financial incentives positively to increased involvement with the community is a creative attempt at consistency with halfway house goals.

Some houses, whether operating within a fixed or within a variable fee system, have tried to keep issues of fees separate from issues of work. Social pressures, expectations and examples provided by staff and by residents act at almost all halfway houses as major incentives to getting and holding jobs—apart from any relations to fees. Some houses attempt to maintain balance between their social service goals and their financial needs by providing "scholarships" at one end of the scale while charging high fees at the other. There are no easy solutions, and halfway houses have so far made no unique contribution to the general problem of fees in relation to services for the mentally disturbed. In many individual cases one has the impression the fee structure was established arbitrarily and without a great deal of thought and that the possibilities of innovation here have received less attention than most areas of halfway house management.

At a conference in May of 1963, representatives of eleven experienced houses suggested that the range of expense for halfway house residence ran roughly between $5 and $11 per person per day. Specific figures depend on many factors, including the comfort and convenience of the house, the services it provides, the number and training of staff, and the size of the resident population. The rough range suggests, however, that, although halfway house costs are not necessarily lower than costs in hospitals which provide principally custodial care, they generally are lower than costs in those hospitals which emphasize programs of treatment.

Although there is a considerable range, the average fee is likely to be low. The $90 median fee can cover expenses only partially, and the questionnaire data indicate that most houses cannot depend on fees for their entire financial support. Table 4 suggests a somewhat bi-modal distribution. Twelve houses indicate that fees cover only 0% to 25% of costs; eleven indicate they cover 75% or more; the median response suggests that fees provide some between 50% and 75% of support. Even so, thirty-three

TABLE 4. Percentage of Costs Covered
by Fees

Percentage	N
0–24	12
25–49	4
50–74	8
75 or more	11
NA[a]	4
No fee	1
	40

[a] Four houses gave no report or said that the question was inapplicable because the house was too newly established to yield any clear indication.

of the houses reporting consider their fees to be adequate; only three consider them inadequate (two of these were about to increase fees). The houses with relatively low fees must obviously depend on other sources of support.

Six of the eleven houses which covered or expected to cover 75% and upwards of their costs through fees were in the group of houses having twenty or more residents; another house felt that it could break even with a resident population of twenty. The break-even point, of course, differs enormously from house to house. Even very high fees may not cover expenses if residents require considerable individual attention from specialized sources and if the house undertakes to provide specialized services.[2] If the resident group is fairly small and considerable professional help is available on the premises, houses must continue to depend on outside sources of income if they are to maintain their standards. If, however, major professional services can be provided under outside auspices, and if the house can encompass a resident population of twenty or more, a halfway house can be self-supporting with rather moderate fees. In early 1963 halfway house workers felt that twenty or more residents, paying something between $125 and $175 a month, would cover basic minimum costs even in an eastern urban setting. The estimate today would probably run somewhat higher.

There are at present houses which manage to maintain themselves entirely out of fees paid by residents or their families, but such houses are few. Only a minority of current halfway house residents are able to pay the higher fees required by houses which are totally self-supporting, and such houses could accommodate only a small proportion of those who might benefit from halfway house residence. Most houses, then, must find auxiliary sources of income.

As to these auxiliary sources, there is once again no clear tradition. Most of the forty halfway houses have received some form of Federal subsidy. Such subsidies are given for short-term purposes of demonstration and research. What to do when the money ends is a serious question. One house became self-supporting by expanding from ten to twenty residents. One house, previously funded as a demonstration project, has turned to the local mental

---

[2] Nor is the need for specialized help necessarily reduced with lesser degrees of disturbance. The resident entering into community life may require guidance, vocational help, psychotherapy more than someone who is not quite ready to engage in the trials of more independent living.

health association for aid. Others may be able to get local subsidies from state, county or city agencies; they may turn to Community Chest, local fund drives, individual donors, and benevolent foundations. What the long-term effects of new affiliations will be on halfway house operations cannot presently be foreseen.

Hospitals too are seldom self-supporting. And it may be that, like hospitals, halfway houses cannot be expected to survive without endowment except in unusual cases. If, however, it can be demonstrated over the next few years that in halfway houses costs are lower than in hospitals with similar rehabilitative aims, and if furthermore it can be shown that halfway house residence results in reduced hospital readmission rates, the obvious benefit to the public will justify continued and increased support of the growing trend to halfway houses.

Yet such figures would tell only a very partial story. The days that someone can be out of a hospital—even if not permanently—are not subject to an easy cost accounting. Nor is it legitimate, even in economic terms, to speak simply of costs. Unlike the hospital patient, the halfway house resident, whether he does volunteer work, or educates himself, or has a paid job, contributes something to the community and adds to its productive power. If he gets paid, he pays taxes. Even if only partially and temporarily, he supports himself. In short, he is a citizen of the community, rather than its ward. And this, too, must be considered in an estimation of costs.

Chapter 7 DEMOGRAPHIC STRUCTURE:
WHO LIVES IN A
HALFWAY HOUSE

THE STRUCTURE OF A HALFWAY HOUSE IS A MORE THAN A MATTER of its physical and administrative features. As we have argued, these are important and they tell much about the differences between mental hospital and halfway house. But as with the mental hospital, the nature of a house—its aims, what it does, and how it does it—will reflect its resident population. This chapter, then, considers who lives in halfway houses.

First, some numbers. All in all, in early 1963, the forty houses served a total of only 483 residents. The average house would thus have 12 residents. Since the average is weighted by those houses which have the larger resident populations, a more accurate picture is given by tabulating number of residents per house (Table 5). As can be seen from the table, the modal house has between 6 and 10 residents; about half have less than 10; a quarter of the houses have between 11 and 15 residents; and slightly over a quarter have more than 15. The maximum number of residents in any one house appears to be about 30, although some facilities seem to have a somewhat larger potential capacity than this. Five houses take 5 or fewer residents; but two of these, we should note, have additional "normal" members.

TABLE 5. Populations of Halfway Houses

	N
5 or less	5
6–10	14
11–15	10
16–20	4
21–30	7
	40

By any criterion, then, most halfway houses are small organizations. This means that, unlike hospitals, the administrative staff structure can be—though it isn't always—relatively simple. (Of this we say more in the next chapter.) It also means that relations among residents, and between staff and residents, are likely to be more immediate, more direct, more personal than in larger organizations. Even if only by virtue of smaller numbers, the halfway house is likely to be more intimate than the hospital ward. At the same time, the halfway house allows for greater privacy than the hospital ward. In most psychiatric wards one is forced to share all private activities with many strangers. Through room arrangements, the halfway house can adapt closeness and distance to the resident's wishes and needs.

Small size is not, however, an unmitigated blessing. In very small groups much is demanded of individual members, and the demands may be too great for a particular resident. The addition of a new member is more likely to precipitate a crisis in a very small group. And although temporary crises may offer valuable potential for learning, the small group is more likely to face permanent total disorganization if it does not exercise careful selection of new members. Furthermore, as we noted earlier, there is the matter of financial viability. For financial independence at reasonable fees a house seems to require an approximate minimum of twenty residents. But since halfway houses emphasize their residential, homelike, atmospheres, adding a number of residents would spoil the atmosphere and be antithetical to the philosophy of the house. One possible compromise is the double-house. These are usually two small houses close to one another, operating under a single administration. There are six such double-houses—that is, six pairs of two houses each—in the sample, and at least one more has developed since the date of the survey.

Those with most experience and most involvement in halfway houses feel strongly that houses should be small enough to avoid an institutional character. The participants in the Conference in May, 1963, felt it would be possible to respond adequately to as many as thirty residents. With thirty it should still be possible to avoid the impersonal atmosphere which results from failure to respond to people as individuals—the identifying mark of an institution. On the other hand, they agreed that houses should avoid having too few residents. With too small a number, static or unmanageably intense relationships and cliques might arise. The ideal number was thought to be one just large enough to permit shifts in relationships as the residents themselves changed.

Where Residents Come From

As might be expected, the residents of halfway houses come predominantly from mental hospitals. Over half the houses (21) received referrals from only a single hospital each; among these were the thirteen Veterans Administration houses. Seven houses received referrals from more than one hospital. The twelve remaining houses found residents more variously: their sources included hospitals, clinics, private practitioners, families and friends.

The direction of movement *from* the hospital *to* the halfway house fits the traditional halfway house emphasis on its function as transition or bridge. So, too, does the fact that the predominant mass of residents, 84%, had been in a mental hospital sometime within the year in which they came to a halfway house. What is strange is that there are others (Table 6). One small group of others (5%) had been hospitalized at one time but had been out of the hospital for between one and five years before coming to the house. These people, then, are making a different use of the halfway house. Instead of bridging the gap between hospital and community, the halfway house provides these residents with a way of maintaining themselves in the community. For this group residence becomes a preventive measure against hospital readmission.

Even more surprising is finding that 46 residents of halfway houses—almost 10% of the sample—have never been hospitalized at all.[1] The number is, of course, small, but that such a class of residents appears in the population at all may suggest a trend toward an alternative use of the halfway house. It represents a way for those undergoing major psychological difficulties to take a partial moratorium from their environment, without completely withdrawing from society. The function of transition between the closed hospital ward and the open community is even more obviously irrelevant here.

Halfway house literature has emphasized rehabilitative functions, but 15% of halfway house residents seem to be using halfway houses as a way to stay out of hospitals and to prevent total alienation from the community.

As such functions become known, halfway houses may be used increasingly as community resources. They may enable those

TABLE 6. Pre-admission Status of Halfway House Residents

Categories	Number of Residents
Never been hospitalized	46
From a hospital within the year	407
Out of a hospital 1 to 5 years before coming	25
Other (another halfway house, special school, etc.)	5
	483

[1] The "normals" living in some halfway houses are excluded from this number.

who are disturbed to maintain a life within the community, avoiding the isolation and the debilitating effects of hospitalization.[2] It is likely that many in treatment at clinics and by private practitioners have family and social lives so disturbed through a variety of circumstances that maintenance of usual patterns of living is grossly interfered with. The halfway house allows a break less than total. At the least, it can serve to allow a partial psycho-social moratorium (Erikson, 1950) for those who need this, while avoiding the noxious effects of long-term hospitalization.

Diagnostic Issues

At present, however, by far the greatest number of halfway house residents have come from mental hospitals, and almost all of the houses were begun with the expectation of serving the needs of such a population. The residents are most likely to have been diagnosed as schizophrenic; there is little difference among halfway houses in the diagnostic labels which were once, or are still, ascribed to their residents.[3] Houses are also generally agreed on their range of exclusions from admission. As a rule, alcoholics and drug addicts are excluded. For these groups special houses have recently been developed (Blacker & Kantor, 1960; Breslin & Crosswhite, 1963), but they are not considered here. Other groups often mentioned as warranting exclusion are those with organic brain defects or severe mental deficiency, overt homosexuals, and those who are likely to show serious anti-social or criminal behavior. The categories of exclusion thus indicate the sensitivities of halfway houses to issues of medical risk, and to issues of major social disruption, both within the resident group and in relation to the social community. Many of the houses ex-

---

[2] At least two houses have made arrangements for the flexible use of hospital resources for immediate and temporary emergencies, a procedure suggestive of Maxwell Jones' use of the hospital as a central resource and emergency facility (Jones, 1953).

[3] Schizophrenia is, of course, the predominant hospital diagnosis for the age group in halfway houses.

cluded such high-risk residents from the outset; others have become more restrictive as a result of difficult experiences. Some houses, however, while excluding these groups at the start, felt that it might be possible later to broaden their admission policies. Candidates for whom there was high social risk might, it was felt, be admitted singly under certain circumstances, if there were a tolerant atmosphere in the house and in the community. The general indications are, however, that living arrangements for those with the more severe social disturbances require separate facilities, or at least a combination of very careful planning and very stable structure.

Apart from their use in determining need for exclusion, specific psychiatric diagnoses seem rather unimportant to most halfway house directors. Eight houses say they prefer residents with similar diagnoses; four others want residents whose diagnoses vary. Three of these latter houses have populations of twenty or more, and one of the possible advantages of the larger house may be to allow for diversity in the resident population. The rest of the forty houses claim diagnosis does not affect their present selection process.

Far more critical for selection than formal diagnosis is the matter of severity of disturbance. Our questionnaire yields only fuzzy clues on this subject, and so long as there is no adequate language for describing severity, comparisons will remain difficult to achieve. Nevertheless, respondents' spontaneous comments about selection and formal reports by halfway houses indicate sharp differences. For example, many respondents note employability as requirement for selection of residents. Such houses are likely to take only those who—either before or shortly after admission to the house—can, with help, find and hold jobs. For other houses, entrance is not contingent on employability. The ability of the resident to get and hold a job is seen rather as one of the end results of successful efforts by the house. What is for some houses a criterion for selection is for others, then, a long-term rehabilitative goal.

Indications of differences in severity of disturbance also

appear, in the few cases where data are available, in average length of hospitalization of residents prior to admission to the house. One may, for example, contrast Conard House (Gumrukcu & Mikels, 1965; Mikels & Gumrukcu, 1963a, 1963b) in San Francisco with Wellmet (Kantor & Greenblatt, 1962) in Boston. The average hospitalization period for ex-patients at Conard House was about 14 months; the average length of hospitalization for ex-patients at Wellmet was 12 years. Conard House, as part of its research program, selects those residents who are good bets for rehabilitation; Wellmet, as part of its research, selects those "considered poor bets for social survival in a community facility, and, inferentially, even poorer bets to maintain themselves independently in a work or other productive role (Conard House Progress Report, 1963; Wellmet Progress Report, 1963)." For most houses the length of previous hospitalization of residents would fall between these two.

Other selective factors enter to create differences in the populations of different halfway houses. Houses dependent on high individual fees can attract residents from upper and middle class socio-economic brackets only. A house sponsored by and responsible to state hospital facilities will, on the other hand, derive its resident population from lower and lower middle class levels. Thus, for example, the average length of education of ex-patients at Conard House, a private organization, is thirteen years. At the State-sponsored Vermont houses, residents have on the average only slightly more than nine years of education. Other divergences in house populations are created by differences in tastes, preferences, interests and motives among those who direct halfway houses. Impersonal factors—location, as noted previously, room arrangement, the size of the resident group, the supervisory structure—will also affect who comes to the house.

Age and Sex in Relation to Structure

Most halfway houses accept candidates of varying ages. The preponderant number of residents are in their twenties and thirties; less than 10% are under twenty years of age, and less than 5% are over 65. Some houses like their resident group to be mixed in age. But there are exceptions, and sometimes, too, other selective factors limit the age range. An example of predetermined selection is a house which is established specifically for young girls; it sets 25 as an upper age limit, and it consciously seeks a homogeneous population. On the other hand, at Wellmet, where there is no attempt to control age variation, the age range is limited by other factors in selection; that is, the choice of the long-term, chronically hospitalized results in an average age of over 45 on admission to Wellmet. A specifically limited age range is likely to impose certain structural features on a house, particularly at the extremes of the range. The house for young girls is, as might be expected, closely supervised, and it has a more than usual number of formal mechanisms for control. A house with many residents over 65 would require special physical and supervisory arrangements.

There is no doubt that existing needs of some age groups are not met by present halfway houses. Partly the problem is one of definition. For example, a house for children would not be known as a halfway house, but rather as a residential treatment center. A halfway house for those over 65 would not suggest transition. Nonetheless, there are gaps at both ends of the age range. Halfway house workers seem particularly cognizant of the need for facilities for adolescents.

Almost twice as many men as women live in halfway houses. This is not surprising when we consider that out of the forty houses, thirteen are sponsored by the Veterans Administration for the care of mostly male war veterans. Nor is it surprising to find that most halfway houses are segregated by sex. Of the forty houses, eighteen are exclusively for men and seven exclusively for women. In this respect most halfway houses are like hospitals where men and women are kept apart.

What is surprising is that fifteen of the forty houses take in both men and women. That this represents innovation is suggested by informal indications (Woodley House Conference, 1963) that each mixed house considers itself unique in this respect and is somewhat surprised to find that there are others. While the mixing of sexes undoubtedly creates some problems, it undoubtedly solves some others. It provides a more natural social atmosphere in the house, and in an area particularly difficult for most residents provides opportunities for social interaction in a somewhat protected environment. Whether the sexes are segregated or mixed unquestionably affects the structural arrangements, including the physical ones, of the house, but our survey yields no specific details on these aspects. The details, and their implications for living arrangements in the rehabilitation of the disturbed, are appropriate material for further study.

"Normals" in Halfway Houses

Five of the forty houses have arrangements whereby, as part of a deliberate plan, "normal" subjects live together in the house with ex-patient residents. Such arrangements are out of the purview of mental hospitals. But they are suited to the halfway house which in its location and physical structure can function simultaneously as a boarding home. The design is most clearly exemplified by Wellmet, where college students serve to bring ex-patients into the house and function as mentors, guides, and co-participants in the living in the house (Umbarger *et al.*, 1962). Another arrangement is that of Conard House which operates primarily as a halfway house but also as an accredited youth hostel. The possibility of the creative use of college students and other volunteers in the living arrangements of the mentally disturbed has appeal to many halfway house directors, and it is likely that this combination, at present rather rare, will be met more frequently in the future.

Halfway house residents, then, form a diverse population, and halfway houses differ in their populations. One is likely to think that on the whole the residents of halfway houses would be less disturbed than the patients in mental hospitals. Yet the participants in the Woodley House Conference of May of 1963 believed that halfway house residents as a group were not markedly different from mental hospital patients in their non-acute periods. The same people, it was felt, may look and behave quite differently in a hospital ward and in a halfway house because of the difference in expectations. Indeed, one participant noted that in actual hospital practice it can happen that while more severely disturbed patients are being discharged, less severely disturbed ones are being admitted. This seemingly contradictory state of affairs can occur when more disturbed patients have reached a so-called point of maximum hospital benefit—the hospital staff has decided it has accomplished all it can; in hospital practice, new and less disturbed patients are more likely to be considered as not yet having had the maximum benefit of hospitalization. Thus, hospitals may have a policy—witting or unwitting—of discharging, where possible, the hopeless and of keeping the hopeful. Surprisingly, then—particularly in contrast to implications in the literature—there seems to be no consensus among halfway-house workers that halfway-house residents are "healthier" than hospital patients.

In summary, a halfway house is likely to have about 10 residents and is unlikely to have more than 30. Most residents are men, between 20 and 30 years of age, who have at one time been labeled as schizophrenic. Houses vary considerably, however, in whom they take: in terms of age, sex, social class and severity of disturbance. In sharp contrast to hospitals, in over a third of the houses residents are not segregated by sex. A small number of houses also have arrangements whereby "normal" people may live in the house and participate in its activities. Surprisingly, there is little evidence or opinion to suggest that as a group halfway house residents differ markedly from mental hospital patients in the severity of psychological disturbance.

Residents are indeed dealt with differently in halfway houses and in hospitals. The use of the term "resident" is not arbitrary. Even in informal discussion, halfway house workers use a variety of terms for those who live in their houses—residents, clients, members, guests, and patients. Where terms other than patient are used, one does *not* have the impression of a euphemism.

Chapter 8   ADMINISTRATIVE
STRUCTURES:
MODELS FOR HALFWAY
HOUSES

In Chapter 2 we spoke of the many recent attempts at
changing the mental hospital. Hopefully, hospitals will continue
to change in the directions suggested by the reports of the Joint
Commission on Mental Illness and Health—in location and size,
in atmosphere, in the vigor of rehabilitative attempts, and in the
development of fully integrated, broadened programs of service
for the mentally disturbed. Perhaps, too, hospitals have reached
the point where they are no longer simply custodians for the in-
curably deranged, and, moreover, where they no longer view
themselves simply as institutional arrangements for achieving the
specific therapist-patient relationship. The teachings of Maxwell
Jones, of Stanton and Schwartz, of the Cummings that hospitals
are social organizations which can be structured to the detriment
or benefit of the rehabilitative process will no doubt be extended.

Hospitals are changing. Yet despite the efforts and daring
which have gone into such changes—and no one who has worked
for any time in a hospital can underestimate these—hospitals remain hospitals. In or out of uniform, doctors, nurses, and attendants remain doctors, nurses, and attendants; they are paid that
way, and they are treated that way—among themselves and by
others. Only very rarely is the primary administrative structure

of the hospital tampered with. For it is, in a large measure, that structure which tells us what a hospital is, and if we no longer had the familiar hierarchies of doctors, nurses, attendants, and patients, we would no longer have a hospital.

It is from this focus that we may turn to look at the staffing patterns of halfway houses. As institutions, halfway houses are too new to have well-established administrative traditions. The very term "halfway house" is in itself ambiguous, implying no particular structure.[1] Halfway is an undefined position, dependent on one's definition of beginning and end points. Similarly, the word house has a broad and ambiguous meaning; a house—as has been noted—is not even necessarily a home. Ambiguity and lack of tradition thus create considerable room for flexibility in the administrative structure of halfway houses (cf. Erikson, Sharp, & Madea, 1963).

Moreover, as we have noted, halfway houses are rather small establishments. Those who work within small organizations identify more strongly with them (Thomas & Fink, 1963), and they participate more fully in them (Barker & Gump, 1964) as compared to members of large organizations. Individual initiative has played a large part in the founding of individual halfway houses, and it plays a large part in their operation. During a period when hospitals have had great difficulty in finding staff, halfway houses have not had much difficulty. One reason may be that halfway house work has some attractions not found in hospitals. In the complex hierarchical organization of a hospital there is little opportunity for a staff person to use his own judgment and his own personal strengths and inclinations or even to manage his own time. Since a halfway house provides these opportunities, staff people are likely to feel a special involvement and interest in their

---

[1] This is untrue for other recent innovations such as day hospitals or night hospitals, although it would hold for something called, let us say, a day center. The word "clinic" also implies a structure, but connotations have been stretched by "beauty clinics," "hair clinics," "foot clinics," etc. The breakdown in meaning is possible because, unlike "hospital," "clinic" does not imply a specific hierarchical staff arrangement. Still, the medical connotations of the term may help determine how such new developments as emergency and suicide clinics are established and run.

work. The requirements and opportunities for individuality would also lead us to expect variety in administrative arrangements.

Variety is immediately apparent if we ask who runs halfway houses. Among the thirteen professionally trained directors involved in day-to-day administration, seven professions are represented. Six of these managing-directors are social workers. But there are also two psychologists, and one each of occupational therapists, vocational rehabilitation counselors, physicians, clergymen, and registered nurses.[2] These data suggest that there is no *specific* professionally based training presently directed toward the management of a halfway house. Nor has there been any investigation of the type of training which would best serve the needs of halfway houses. Although the predominant single profession among trained directors is social work, interest and initiative seem to be the primary selective forces, and these may derive from a variety of disciplines.

Given individual and professional diversity, and a definition with the main characteristic of ambiguity, it is hard to generalize about administrative structure. The staffs of halfway houses vary considerably both in number and in kind and amount of training. In size alone they vary from a single owner–manager to the numerous, almost "family-type" staffs of the large rural house. A simple scheme for categorizing is suggested by the questionnaires. In almost two-thirds (27) of the houses the immediate supervisory personnel are nonprofessionals; in the remaining third immediate supervisors are professionally trained. We look, first, at this difference but our primary interest is in its overlap with another, less explicit difference—that between traditional medically oriented and innovative nonmedical administrative styles.

Nonprofessionally versus Professionally Managed Houses

One criterion for the selection of the sample was that, in order to be defined as a halfway house, the house must maintain

[2] Non-registered nurses of whom there are several are considered in the nonprofessional category.

something of a professional orientation. This criterion eliminated the more informal types of boarding houses from the study. Thus, all forty houses have some association with professional personnel. The form of association varies, however. Some houses are directly staffed by professional personnel; others employ professionals solely in an advisory or consultant capacity.

As noted, in almost two-thirds of the houses immediate supervisors are nonprofessionals. Such nonprofessional staff often have a background of interest in and work with people—nursing, volunteer work with groups, running a boarding house. They usually have a benevolent interest in psychiatric rehabilitation. Those who own a boarding house which they lend to these purposes can combine such interests with their wish to use their premises fully. But the association of the nonprofessional with the house *as* a halfway house more often follows than precedes conceptualization and development of the facility. That is, it is professionals who conceive of the initial idea, plan the policies, and then go about searching for a suitable nonprofessional director. Although the nonprofessional director has major responsibility for day-to-day management and may be in that sense the functional head of house operations, he is not necessarily the nominal director, nor is he likely to play a primary role in the determination of policy.

The houses which do not have professionally trained people living and working on the premises have a close working association with a professional organization or with one or more individual professionals. Such professional staff is generally not associated primarily with day-to-day management, although it may set initial policies and consult on changes. In some cases formal arrangements exist for periodic staff meetings between professional staff and nonprofessional managers for discussing problems of the house or of individual residents. Sometimes arrangements are less formal, with residents visiting individual therapists at a hospital or in the community, and with periodic consultation between such therapists and the nonprofessional house director.

In the nonprofessionally managed houses the actual functioning director is often administratively subordinate to the occasional consultant. What characterizes such houses is an administrative arrangement involving a professional and most often superordinate director and/or consultant, and a nonprofessional and probably subordinate house manager. The professionals do not live on the premises, though they may be involved in house management policies in varying degrees. The house manager maintains the day-to-day process, but may not be responsible for the policies by which the house is run.

In about one-third of the houses there is a professionally trained director involved in day-to-day administration on the premises. We have already commented on the diversity of professions represented among the professional directors. Despite this diversity a consistency in style of operation seems to emerge. In contrast to the nonprofessional management in which life within the house is seen as somewhat peripheral to change in the residents, the professionally managed house tends to view its structure as playing a fundamental part in effecting change.

These differences in viewpoints are not invariably associated with the professional-nonprofessional dichotomy. There are ambiguities in classification and there are also some outstanding exceptions. For example, Spring Lake Ranch is not professionally managed if we limit our definition to the traditional mental health professions. Nonetheless, its program is designed to effect changes and to rehabilitate its residents by means of the kind of life they participate in, as organized and structured by the staff. Again, Woodley House, although managed by two highly experienced and skilled occupational therapists, prides itself on its deprofessionalization and at times claims that the house is nothing more than a "good place to live for those who like to live there." Despite these claims, or rather lack of claims, house policies and activities represent a sophisticated approach to teaching people how to live better lives. Perhaps, instead of the professional-nonprofessional classification we might more usefully have differentiated between those houses which are dependent on external hierarchical control and those which are relatively independent. But the questionnaire, as designed, does not enable us to do this. Clearly the houses which are professionally managed are somewhat more likely to be independent and to develop innovative styles in contrast to the traditionally oriented styles of less independent, nonprofessionally managed halfway houses. It is to the difference between these approaches to dealing with the mentally disturbed that we now turn.

Traditional versus Innovative Styles

The orientation of nonprofessionally managed halfway houses is likely to favor a traditional psychiatric point of view. The traditionally oriented house views its residents as individual psychiatric patients. Indeed, it terms its residents *patients,* and it is their problems as patients which are emphasized. The house is primarily a place to live while the important "treatment" goes on elsewhere —with outside therapists, social workers, vocational counselors. The house may be a rather special place to live: it may maintain a more than usual sensitivity to the needs and to the pathology of its individual residents. It may also be special in providing a high degree of support and control for those residents who need it, and it may provide and encourage an active social life for those who might otherwise be isolated. Special techniques, such as group therapy, may even be brought into the house. But the life that goes on *within* the house is seen as secondary. Except during individual crises which require special consideration and treatment, the structural arrangements of the house and the processes of life within it are not subject to continuous thought and review. The halfway house itself is not emphasized as a major agent for significant change in people's lives.

The orientation of the professionally managed house is more likely to deviate from the traditional psychiatric emphasis on the individual patient. The deviation is likely to be a conscious one. As we noted previously, it is reflected in terms used, rather unselfconsciously and non-euphemistically, for house populations—residents, clients, guests.

These innovatively oriented houses tend to see themselves and their activities as specific agents for change. They are likely to be sensitive to structural patterns of interpersonal relations within the house as a whole, and they may consciously plan arrangements and activities so as to bring about group and individual change. As examples, the inclusion of normal residents within the house group, the initiation of procedures for self-management by the residents, the introduction of mixed groups of men and women residents are seen as planned steps toward the residents' assumption of life in the broader community.

Moreover, crisis tends to be looked upon as more than an individual disruption to be dealt with on a momentary basis; it may be seen as indicative of group processes within the house. That is, although individual pathology is recognized, the crisis event is not seen solely as an outburst of individual pathology. It may rather become the occasion for re-examination and revision of house policies and functions.

Perhaps the most dramatic example of innovative design is represented by Wellmet (Kantor & Greenblatt, 1962; Kantor & Gelineau, 1963; Umbarger et al., 1962). As noted earlier, the house membership at Wellmet is composed of former mental hospital patients and of normal college students. Ex-patients, both male and female, were hospitalized an average of twelve years before coming to the house. As part of a volunteer program, college students worked in the hospital setting with these patients on an intensive one-to-one basis; if and when these students felt that the patients were ready, they argued for bringing them into the house as residents (Dohan, 1957).

The students are volunteers rather than professionals. Wellmet does *not* have a professional person as manager on the premises, and the omission is intentional since the house is designed to function as a cooperative. "The student residents are advised and supervised by an outside professional staff including a vocational rehabilitation counselor, a social worker, and a psychiatrist. Along with nonresident students they conduct a program in this cooperative living milieu which is aimed at achieving the social, psychological, and vocational rehabilitation of the patients (Kantor & Gelineau, 1963)."

The basic premise underlying Wellmet's organization is that the social system of which the chronic patient is a member makes major impact upon his progress. The Directors feel that ". . . the large public mental hospital, particularly as it is exemplified in the chronic ward where treatment facilities are at a minimum or non-existent, acts to sustain pathology, increase chronicity, and block any potential for rehabilitation that the patient retains (Kantor & Gelineau, 1963)." Among the factors in hospitals inhibiting resocialization, Kantor and Gelineau list the rigid social controls, the impermeable status hierarchies, the degradation rituals imposed on patients, the sharp restriction of roles and role partners, and the insulation from the influences and demands of ordinary society. "These and other mechanisms," Kantor and Gelineau suggest, "hold the psychotic in the role of chronic patient."

With this view as a starting point, Wellmet's emphasis is on the house as a social system. The attempt is to develop a new system which is specifically directed toward creating social processes differing from those in the hospital. The social milieu, specific social schema and modes of interaction are continuously modified through conscious periodic maneuvers. The periodic modifications are geared not only to the rehabilitative process for the ex-patients as a group, but are at times designed to enhance the progress of a specific individual. In a later section we give a brief illustration of this procedure.

Wellmet's program is unique, and few if any other halfway houses have a so systematically social-psychological approach. Yet each of the innovatively oriented houses views itself, more or less explicitly, as a social system, and as one which contrasts with that of the mental hospital. We have already noted some comments by Woodley House about the problems of hospital reform (Rothwell & Doniger, 1963). Rothwell and Doniger comment critically on attempts to introduce artificially into the hospital setting features which are natural and unaffected in a halfway house.

They suggest that the simple, non-authoritarian organization of the halfway house is a function of its size and staff orientation, and that ". . . the deliberate abandonment of all the usual hospital-like controls is possible only because the halfway house is not medically supervised (p. 285)."[3] As an example, they comment—as do the directors of Wellmet—on the differences between the identity definitions of people in halfway houses as compared to hospitals. "When a Woodley House resident said, 'I'm not an artist, I'm a patient,' he was told that he was a patient an hour a day, when he saw his doctor, but that he could not be a patient the other 23 hours . . . the staff continued to resist his attempts to be treated like and have the privileges of a patient. In hospitals the argument is often reversed and conflict arises because the patients will not assume patient roles so that the staff can practice its helping role (p. 285)." Unlike the situation in hospitals, in a halfway house ". . . the residents and staff live in the same world and the staff has no real power over residents' lives. Like the staff members, residents have jobs and occasionally have positions on a par with or of higher status than staff members. They go to the same theaters and shop in the same stores. At home they cook in the same kitchen, eat in the same dining room, and share the same bathrooms. Having so much in common with the residents and so few situations which might perpetuate distance from them, the staff finds that its ability to consider residents as peers rather than patients is fostered (p. 286)." The authors emphasize that not only differences in philosophy, but also differences in structure affect the relationships between staff and residents.

We have noted Jules Henry's comments about multiple subordination patterns characteristic of hospital structures, and we have noted some of the complications induced by these patterns Doniger, Rothwell, and Cohen (1963) contrast this with the administrative pattern of simple undifferentiated subordination that characterizes Woodley House:

[3] They add that, "This permits alteration of the legal and ethical responsibilities of supervision (p. 285)."

Woodley House is now run as a partnership, by its director (Joan Doniger) and her associate, Edith Maeda, with occasional assistance from graduate students. We have no fixed hours of duty. Instead, like mothers, we live such a sensible day that we often cannot tell when we're working; we may do personal laundry at Woodley House but worry about its problems when we are at home. At Woodley House our tasks are mixed: cooking, writing papers, cleaning the basement. We do all kinds of work, because we like it and because we think it's important. When people ask, "Aren't you looking forward to the day when you have a lot of money and don't have to do the cooking?," we answer that if we had a lot of money we'd still do the cooking, because the kitchen is where many good things happen. Also, we are trying to sell our residents on the idea that work of all kinds has dignity, and it is easier to do this if we work ourselves. Moreover, chores are tension reducing. It's hard to sit and listen to someone tell you she is going to kill herself, but if you're making supper and ask her to help, it does water the problem down.

. . . Since there are only two staff members, we have no meetings, no checking with higher authorities, no supervision of lower-level workers, nor even much incentive to coordinate our activities once we have decided who will work when. Each of us is independent. In this setup, residents' problems emerge with undreamed-of clarity, and we can react with appropriate speed. Tensions don't build up as they do in hospitals, and those which do can be dissipated more easily than on a hospital ward. We can walk out, the residents can walk out, or one of us can make coffee or bake a cake or go to bed.

It is also easier in our setting than in hospitals to keep communication simple. When Mary complained that Barbara's cat used her cat's kitty litter and wanted us to speak to Barbara about it, we aid, "Tell her yourself." We have had people who, we were warned, had been extremely manipulative patients; they had long records of setting nurse against nurse, doctor against nurse, one shift against the other. But they lacked opportunity for this in Woodley House (p. 194).

There is a disarming and somewhat deceptive simplicity in the above description. Yet it is startlingly innovative in its attempt to cut through the complexities created by more medically oriented approaches. Two professional occupational therapists are responsible for the day-to-day management of Woodley House.

Both have a rich background in work with disturbed adults and children. It might seem then that the conscious deprofessionalization and the disclaimers of formal treatment procedures represent something of a paradox. But such views as Woodley House represents arise not through lack of skills. On the contrary, they result from deliberate attempts to utilize the knowledge derived from many years of professional experience. Only on the basis of such experience could the directors divorce themselves from nonfunctional trivia and attend to the parameters of the tasks at hand. The patterns of interaction which evolve from the Woodley House structure are in one sense simple, but, as we show more fully later, they imply the skills and the sophistication required for dealing optimally with the events of daily experience.[4]

Administrative Boards

A help and safeguard in the administration of halfway houses are advisory or managing boards or committees. In some cases boards were active in the founding of the house; in other cases they were a later development. About half the houses ($N=22$) have formal boards. Only four houses are without a board of any sort.[5]

How active the board is and how wide the range of decisions it becomes involved in varies greatly from house to house. Much depends on the size of the house staff and its training. In houses which are adequately staffed the board may take little or no active role in determining the way the house functions. Where

---

[4] Fritz Redl discusses this topic in terms of what he has called the "life space interview (Redl, 1959a)."

[5] Houses sponsored by the Veterans Administration do not have formal boards. In all but one of these houses there is collaboration between the house parent or "sponsor," as he or she is frequently termed, and Veterans Administration social workers and psychiatrists. The relation is such that the primary hospital referring source constitutes a policy board, although it is not designated as such. One Veterans Administration house was originally founded by a charitable institution and preserves the board arrangement worked out at that time.

staff is in a sense marginal—through pressure of time, inadequate training, personal inadequacies—the role of the board in decision making is increased. Houses which are nonprofessionally managed are more likely to have active boards, in which professionals play a major part in policy decisions (Lyman, 1961).

Thus, for most houses, decision making is a divided function. Both professionals and nonprofessional resident-managers must make day-to-day decisions, but policy decisions generally revert to a board or committee. Whether the board makes minor as well as major decisions will depend on its constitution, and that constitution will vary with the orientation, the structure, and the staffing of the halfway house.

Definition of policy is not the only board function, although it is the most traditional one. Boards may be selected, for example, to provide a pool of resource people who can serve as specialists in a number of areas pertinent to the administration of the house. Because of the nature of problems which halfway houses may meet, it is useful to have lawyers, accountants, psychiatrists, other physicians, industrialists, and legislators represented on the board. Such members can be called upon for advice in the area of their specialties. Their services are often at no cost to the house, and, in donating these services, they are able to supply a fuller understanding of the house and its goals than would be possible for outside professionals. Sometimes wives are appointed in lieu of the specialists themselves. These women can obtain professional help when necessary, and they may be able to devote more interest to the house than would their professional husbands.

Boards may also play a critical role in fund raising. Experienced civic leaders, familiar with people and organizations in the community, can be most useful in obtaining or supplementing the financial support of the house. Moreover, such people can serve the vital function of bringing knowledge of the halfway house to the community and of the community to the halfway house, and in mediating between the house and the broader community. Such functions form a part of the tasks of any board. Whether a board is composed of high-ranking mental health professionals, of specialists in diverse areas of administration, of social and community leaders, or of all three, it plays a major role in legitimization of the house. It indicates a measure of respectability, solvency, and competency. Such legitimization is particularly important for new and nontraditional institutions like the halfway house.

Most of the board functions noted above are suggested in an informal description by Susan Lyman, President of the Board of Rutland Corner House:

> A word about the Board of Managers, and their role in the development of the experiment. First of all, who are they? Essentially, a lay group: mothers of families; a few grandmothers; college graduates for the most part; a couple of social workers; an architect; a couple with business training; these all women. For men: two lawyers and two bankers. The Board of Managers meets once a month to hear reports on activity at the House and to make policy, the latter for the most part at the recommendation of an Executive Committee working with staff. No psychiatrists on the Board, you ask? No, because the professional service our residents need is graciously supplied by the Massachusetts Mental Health Center. We do have, however, *Mrs.* Harry Solomon [Ed.: the wife of a prominent Boston psychiatrist].

> Second point about the Board of Managers: it has seen to the sound and successful handling of the agency's invested capital for 83 years, so that today the House corporation is solvent, and with an income of approximately $14,000 per annum, financially independent of public—state or city—and private community chest organizations. Financial independence allows the Board of Managers considerable latitude in policy-making, a prerogative it treasures.

> Third: the fact that the Board of Managers in a real sense represents the community and acts as a community sounding-board for what is acceptable and helped stabilize the development of the experiment. Let me give you an example here: one girl, a resident of the House, wanted to drive other residents about in her automobile while she was staying at the House. Unbeknownst to her companions, she was subject to epileptic seizures. This inevitably presented a certain hazard to other residents, with the possibility of the type of incident the lay Board wishes to avoid until the halfway house movement is quite secure. The Board said no.

> And last but most: the Board of Managers is responsible for the staff of the agency (Lyman, 1961, pp. 81–82).

Part

III

OPERATIONS

THE LITERATURE ON HALFWAY HOUSES UNIVERSALLY REFERS TO their transitional function. So do almost all questionnaire respondents. Most often they state explicitly that the halfway house is designed to function as a bridge between mental hospital and community, and where this statement is not overt it is implied. Clearly then, most houses accept as a value the notion of the patient's rehabilitation to life in its typical community aspects. Still, while they are rather rare, there appear to be some exceptions to this orientation. The exceptions tend to occur in the rural houses and the religiously oriented ones and in only a few of these. But these few do not emphasize the transitional function. They seem less concerned with having the resident get back to his former community than with providing a gratifying life within the halfway house itself, and sometimes what might be thought of as a spiritual reorientation. But aside from these few exceptions, the major functional premise is that the halfway house resident is to be brought into closer relation with the pattern of living in ordinary communities.

Some hints of how halfway houses go about reaching this goal have been suggested in the previous chapters on structure. In contrast to mental hospitals, halfway houses are located predominantly in urban residential areas; they remain small, and emphasize a homelike atmosphere; a fair proportion of houses includes both men and women, and a number even include "normals" among their residents.

The structural features provide a foundation. To see more than this foundation and move beyond the vague generalization of "transition" or "bridge," it is necessary to ask how halfway houses operate. Such a question can be answered fully only by an intimate detailing of precisely what goes on from the time a potential resident is being considered as a house member until the time he leaves. Such operational detail is clearly beyond the scope of a questionnaire survey. Nonetheless, we can become at least somewhat better acquainted with actual modes of operation by surveying what halfway houses say they do. The following chapters consider some aspects of the transactions between house and resident. The *caveat* should be borne in mind, however, that one is dealing with the actualities of functioning only in so far as these are reflected in the stated judgments and attitudes of the respondents, who are the staff and not the residents of halfway houses. It is likely that the judgments and attitudes reflect to some degree what halfway houses actually do, but to what degree is unknown.

Chapter 9   THE TASKS OF HALFWAY
HOUSES; THE NEW RESIDENT

Selecting the New Resident

CHAPTER 7 DESCRIBED SOME CHARACTERISTICS OF THE RESIDENTS
of halfway houses and some of the criteria which halfway houses
use in selecting residents. Here our concern is primarily with operating procedures in selection and admission of the new resident.

Although the questionnaire does not inquire about details
of the admission process, brochures and informal discussions suggest that one finds here again the considerable diversity which
characterizes halfway houses. Most houses have, however, some
formal established procedure for application and admission. When
the house is closely associated with a single hospital, as are Veterans
Administration houses and some others, a committee of the hospital staff will most often do the primary screening and selection.
Sometimes there is more than one committee, and hospital screening and selection is followed by a formal gating procedure through
a committee composed of the professionals directly associated with
the house. A rather typical formal admission program is described
by Gutman House:

> A patient considered for referral to the house is called to the at-
> tention of the in-hospital Screening Committee. This committee is

composed of the project psychiatrist, and other staff members representing all of the hospital disciplines. They provide the initial screening of patients to assess readiness for and feasibility of referral to the rehabilitation house. Their primary role is to evaluate those patients who are judged to be in need of a transitional facility and specifically the services provided by the rehabilitation house. This committee then makes its recommendation that the patient's case be presented to the house Admissions Committee or for continuation in the inhospital rehabilitation program.

Criteria for selection has been broadly defined in order that there may be more latitude in exploring all of the possible needs which could be met by the rehabilitation house. General criteria have been established, however, in order to provide a frame of reference for the initial selection of house residents. Status is thus evaluated in the following areas: stability of the psychosis, reality orientation, participation in the in-hospital rehabilitation program, emergence of realistic vocational and social planning.

When a patient is considered by the in-hospital screening committee to be a feasible candidate for referral to the house his case is called to the attention of the admissions committee. This committee is composed of the project psychiatrist for each of the state mental hospitals, the project social worker, and the project rehabilitation counselor. (This is the professional staff . . . and its function as an admissions committee is only one of [its] many roles.)

This committee is responsible for total evaluation of each patient presented to them. The patient's status mentally, physically, socially, and vocationally is thoroughly reviewed. Feasibility of the patient's admission as a resident of the house is the central theme. This committee has the final authority and responsibility for decision regarding the needs which determine referral, the nature and degree of services. A screening information summary is prepared by the in-hospital Screening Committee and this serves as the guide for evaluation by the Admissions Committee. Evaluation is concerned with the patient's potential employability, readiness to leave the hospital, and readiness to accept referral to the rehabilitation house. When a patient is considered by the committee to be a feasible candidate for residency, the hospital is notified of the patient's acceptance and planning for his admission takes place. Normally the residents are admitted within one week following evaluation by the Admissions Committee . . .

Several days prior to the resident's admission, the rehabilitation counselor presents a summary of the case to the housemanagers. This discussion centers around the needs of the resident and provides for the housemanagers some insights into his problems. When the resident arrives the housemanagers welcome him to the house. He is assigned to his room, introduced to fellow residents and is given a copy of the house rules (Gutman House Progress Report, 1963).

Formal mechanisms such as those above are apt to be adopted by traditionally oriented houses with nonprofessional house managers. In sharp contrast are the informal admission procedures of a few houses. An example is Woodley House:

Residents find their way to our House through many paths. Sometimes a relative or friend calls first, more often a physician. But [each resident is] sponsored by a therapist, a hospital, or an agency who will continue to see him as long as he is in the House . . . One of the secrets of our success has been a loose intake policy. If the prospect has a therapist, and we have space, we take him (Doniger, 1964).

There is no admission procedure beyond an informal threeway discussion with the therapist, patient, and either the director or her associate, in which mutual expectations and obligations are discussed, and in which the staff member emphasizes the lack of controls and the lack of protection that such controls might have offered the residents in prior institutions . . . Woodley House receives no case histories. The referring therapist is asked only what he thinks is the best and the worst which might happen to the patient who is moving to the house (Rothwell & Doniger, 1963, pp. 282–283).

Even when the selection process is highly formalized according to official dicta, one has the impression that the procedures are not quite as tight as they may seem, and that many informal considerations may enter into choice of resident. Certainly, the prospective candidate's desire to move into the house is essential to his being accepted. Furthermore, committees responsible for admission, if they are knowledgeable about the house, will in their review consider a number of factors having to do not only with the applicant's presenting characteristics but also with the structure of the house. For example, although the screening for Rutland Corner House is done primarily by the hospital from which the applicant comes, Landy notes a number of additional questions which the hospital and the House explore with each candidacy: "(1) Is there room? (2) Who seems neediest—in terms of personal means, rehabilitation potential and community resources and opportunities? (3) Will she fit into the existing group—in terms of age, temperament and special behavior problems? A candidate rejected at one point in time may be acceptable at another—and vice versa. (4) Does the House director deem the candidate a desirable member and one with whom there seems a reasonable probability of establishing congenial social relations (Landy, 1961, pp. 96–97)."

Chance factors, personal predilections, social and individual influences also weigh in the informal aspects of the admission process. Doniger comments on these issues:

> Chance—that is, applying at a time when someone is leaving—has a lot to do with admission. We are influenced by pressure from sponsors. A doctor who calls and talks enthusiastically about his patient gets more attention than one who writes a formal note. We also try to keep the group balanced and mixed. For example, we keep the ages and sexes mixed so that if we have too many young people or too many men, we take somebody older or choose a woman; if there are too many non-workers, we'll only take somebody with a job; if there are too many depressed people, we'll take somebody a little manicky; if too many people are talking Aristotelian logic, we look for a comic-book reader (Doniger, 1964).

It is surprising, in view of the anti-authoritarian, anti-hierarchial emphasis on the halfway house movement, that the residents have so little part in the formal process of choosing a new member. So far as we know, only in one house, Wellmet, do the residents have a major role in deciding on an applicant. Although there is an initial screening team of psychiatric, sociological and vocational personnel which reviews all referrals, the final decision at Wellmet is made by mutual agreement of house members—both ex-patients and college student volunteers—with professional staff playing little or no part in the process. And probably the attitudes of the members of other halfway houses do exercise an informal influence in the selection of a prospective candidate. For, unlike mental hospitals, halfway houses encourage new applicants to visit before admission. Thus, before the mutual choice of house and resident is made, the new candidate has the opportunity to interact with the house members, and they have the opportunity to interact with him. Because of the easy informal communication between the staff and residents of halfway houses, it is likely that attitudes toward the applicant are conveyed to the staff. To what extent the decision-making members of the staff are influenced by the views of house members is unknown, but informal patterns of influence are effected through such visits.

Orientation and Introduction

Most halfway houses (34 of the 40) encouraged residents to visit before admission; only two did not encourage such visits, and four houses did not reply to the questionnaire item. All of the houses which invited prospects to visit said that some or many do actually come. Some houses make special efforts along this line, and three make such visits a mandatory prerequisite for admission. One house, for example, requires that the prospective candidate visit the house for at least an entire weekend, and preferably for two or three, before making the decision. Another house maintains what might be thought of as an extended visiting program, since residents are accepted on a trial basis for the first two months of their stay and continuing residence is contingent on evaluation procedures at the end of each month. On the other hand, rural houses, since they are remote and visiting them requires considerable travel and expense, seldom have advance visits whether or not these are encouraged.

Houses which are closely associated with a particular hospital may complete much of the orientation of prospective residents while the latter are still in the hospital. The task of liaison is often undertaken by a hospital social worker who describes the halfway house and its customs to the candidate. An example of an especially effective hospital orientation program is that of the Vermont Rehabilitation Houses, based on their close association with the State Hospital: candidates for the two halfway houses are placed on a separate hospital ward where they can gradually begin to assume some of the freedoms and responsibilities they will be expected to deal with on moving into a halfway house.

When the prospective resident comes to the house to visit or/join the group, a more specific discussion is likely to take place with the house manager or a staff person, who outlines patterns of life at the house and tells the candidate what he can expect and what will be expected of him should he come. A fairly typical description is given by Gomness, Director of Rutland Corner House:

> . . . the patient makes an appointment to visit the house and we spend an hour or more together discussing the house, group living, her general interests, future plans, and try to find some common interest on which to fashion a relationship between us. Sometimes there are two or three such visits and occasionally a prospective candidate has dinner with us which gives her an opportunity to meet the other members of the household and for the group in the house to meet a possible new member (Gomness, 1961, p. 86).

Once the new resident enters the house as a member, there is little likelihood that he will be lost, as is the case on a large hospital ward. In the halfway house he joins a small number of people and his presence is noticeable. The staff may actively encourage social relations with the new member, or—as at Gutman House—it may deliberately keep contact minimal during the first few days after admission, leaving the resident free to feel out his new environment at his own pace. In either case, introductions are natural and the living and dining arrangements promote a simple and gradual entree into the life of the house.

Chapter 10 LIVING IN THE HOUSE:
CODES FOR RESIDENTS

Mental Hospital and Halfway House

EVERY SOCIETY HAS CODES WHICH DEFINE FOR ITS MEMBERS desirable and undesirable actions. In our own society some codes are expressed in the form of written rules and regulations—as with laws, building and traffic regulations. Most codes of behavior are, however, unwritten. We learn them in childhood through the process of socialization by which the preservers of social norms —our parents—teach us what is appropriate and what is inappropriate. Even such rules as are written are seldom read except by experts in such matters, and we learn mostly through informal communication and observation.

We need not here be especially concerned with the mechanics of such learning. Several points, however, require comment. First is the fact that there are sanctions—rewards and penalties—established by societies for conforming or breaking with their social codes. The sanctions not only implement learning but must themselves be learned. They, too, are mostly unwritten and are incorporated informally—along with the codes to which they refer—in the process of growing up.

Another point is that in a complex society such as ours codes and sanction systems are not the same throughout the society.

That is, although some rules are common to all members of a society, particular subgroups will have their own systems of rules and modes of enforcement. Not only do we find class differences, but also differences among ethnic and occupational subgroups and even from family to family within a particular subgroup. The existence of such differences means that new learning is constantly required in negotiating the transitions of a differentiated yet mobile society.

Apart from the divisions made by regional, social, economic ethnic and familial differences are the differentiations which exist within any system of codes. Learning seldom consists of total prescriptions and injunctions. The "thou shalts" and the "thou shalt nots" of a society are allocated according to particular status —social or developmental—and to particular times and places. Examples are obvious enough. Behavior acceptable in a five year old is unacceptable in a ten year old; manner and tone of voice distinguish friends from strangers—even reflect the status of the stranger—and they are varied to suit various occasions—to a ball game, an intimate social gathering, a funeral. Even the injunction against killing is countermanded under conditions of war. Thus, what we must learn in the course of development is not so much, for example, to avoid dependency or aggressivity—any more than we learn to avoid urination—but rather the time, place and circumstances which render dependence or aggression appropriate or inappropriate. Moreover, not only is what we learn tailored to fit time, place and social context, but sanctions tend to be similarly localized. Only for very young children are the rewards and punishments of one sphere of life wholly transferable to other spheres. That is—as we noted earlier, following Goffman (1961)—in ordinary adult life in a complex differentiated society, the sanction systems of family, occupational, social and recreational life are kept somewhat apart from one another; accomplishments and successes or misdeeds and failures in one area of life do not inevitably affect other areas.

A final point to be noted here is that there are always discrepancies between a society's overt codes—whether these are written or unwritten—and the actualities of what is accepted or unaccepted. Such gaps are in part due to changes in mores and customs and to a generational lag, whereby it becomes inevitable in a rapidly changing society that children will be taught rules which are already partly outmoded. But gaps exist also because overt codes tend to represent idealized, simplified and institution-alized versions of right and wrong. In actual life there is in most social codes some measure of leeway. Such leeway allows for what Goffman speaks of as *secondary adjustments,* the unauthorized arrangements by which members of organizations get around, stand apart from, and even "work" the organization's assumptions as to what members should do and what they should be. One who conformed consistently and completely with overt societal rules would be as conspicuous in his compulsivity as one who always obeys grammatical rules is by his pedantry. Acceptable—though unofficial—deviations and their limits must also be learned. In this sense we all learn, more or less, to "con" the systems we live in.

In the total institution the rights and privileges of ordi-nary social life are abrogated. The inmate enters into a system which is—unless he has previously been a member of a total institution—utterly new and strange. In the mental hospital he must learn to do without the accoutrements of ordinary existence —his own clothes, pocket money, matches, a watch, a place for personal belongings. He must learn new codes and standards— "good" and "bad" wards, the behaviors associated with them, the system of transfer in the hospital, the tone and manner of a patient with attendants, nurses, psychiatrists. The rights of ordinary citi-zens become the incentives of the total institution; the inmate must learn a system of rewards and penalties whereby possession of cigarettes and matches, making common purchases, shaving oneself, some choice over one's work and one's companions, ordi-nary freedom of movement and social intercourse become special privileges to be granted or removed. He must learn that no action of his fails to be subject to that single system and that a gesture toward an attendant on the ward can affect his work assignment or his presence at a social function. With brilliance and compassion Goffman (1961) describes the wondrously detailed under-life which develops in these circumstances. One may indeed question, with him, whether those inmates who adjust most adequately to the system can, after a long enough term, be at all capable of entering ordinary society.

Halfway houses have not yet severed their connections with the hospital model. That this is so is quite natural, since the halfway house is generally seen as a way-station in the career of the "sick" or "convalescing" patient. But because it deals in transition, the halfway house cannot be a total institution. That is, if it is to meet its ostensible functions, it must forego total control over the lives of its residents and relegate some measure of control to the various sanction systems of the ordinary community.

Summaries of written and unwritten rules for residents, difficulties with and changes in such rules, and methods of enforcement of rules were requested in the questionnaire (see APPENDIX A, p. 320). The responses to these items cannot, of course, give us the details of day-to-day life in a particular house, but they do convey something of the atmosphere. And again, in the approaches of the forty houses which constitute the sample, one finds similarities, but mostly marked variety. The number of rules, their nature, and how they are expressed differ radically from house to house.

Written and Unwritten Rules

There is no question that halfway houses have rules. Like all arrangements where people are close enough to interact with one another, and where a common basis for expectation and prediction is required, halfway houses operate according to codes. But like private homes, the great majority of halfway houses do not feel a need for *written* rules. Of the forty houses only thirteen said they had written rules and one house was about to change this at the time of the questionnaire, sensing that their written rules were "too impersonal, tend toward regimentation, and are too much like the situation in the hospital setting." Four houses, which lacked written rules, comment explicitly that their rules are "natural," "common," or "ordinary" ones. For example: "Our house rules are all the rules of common sense, safety, courtesy and morality by conventional, middle-class standards, and if you need to find out what they are, all you have to do is break one;" from another house: "Residents are expected to conform to the standards of the community and of society."

Those who defend written rules speak of their residents' needs for structure. They argue that residents need to know very clearly what is expected of them, and that by removing some ambiguity from the living situation, they simplify life and provide security for the still handicapped person. One house points to its experience: when written rules were abolished—as an experiment —residents requested their reinstatement. A further, more subtle argument in favor of written rules is a variation on the structure theme: explicit rules constitute a testing ground; even if they are broken on occasion, they serve as a background against which one can delineate oneself.

In the general community many rules are commonly understood, but few are written down. So it is with most halfway houses. Unwritten rules may produce ambiguity, but proponents believe such ambiguity is realistic: the resident has to learn to adjust to the kind of world he will face on leaving the house. Written rules, they feel, encourage a dependence on others for defining and limiting behavior and fail to maximize the potentialities for learning which a halfway house can offer. The proponents of ambiguity suggest that in a halfway house the resident can benefit from the opportunity for learning to adjust to a setting resembling those in the broader community, but where the penalties for infraction of commonly understood social customs are less harsh.

One might expect that houses whose residents are more severely disturbed would favor the structure of written rules, and that houses whose residents are less disturbed would favor the ambiguity of unwritten codes. But no such general pattern emerges from the questionnaires. Whether the rules of a house are written or oral, highly explicit or vague, seems to have, in practice, little to do with the psychiatric status of its residents. Thus, a house composed of members selected for their high rehabilitation potential seems as likely (or unlikely) to have written rules as one composed of ex-long-term hospital patients. Factors other than psychiatric status seem relevant here. For example, a house for young adolescent girls presents to new residents a brochure of highly explicit written rules: apparently the management feels obligated to act in place of parents. At some other houses written rules have evolved, not from management, but by the decisions of the residents themselves. There is a tendency, commented on by several respondents, for more established houses to minimize or drop their written rules after a time.

Rules, Proscriptions, Requirements

Even those houses which are careful *not* to spell out a list of *do's* and *don'ts* on paper have certain restrictions which they feel are vital to the functioning of the house and which are soon made explicit to the new resident. Most common are the general codes which relate to communal living. Thus one finds that most of the rules are similar to those of boarding homes or residential hotels for single men or women. Restrictions are made on noise —for example, loud playing of radios, television, phonographs is prohibited after ten or eleven p.m.; one house comments that such rules simply reflect city ordinances. Another rule for general convenience is that residents are encouraged to come to meals on time or to inform staff in advance of their absence. In the same general class we may include a few rules which are more specifically personal but still are fairly common in middle-class boarding houses. Almost all houses mention some restriction of the use of alcohol; most prohibit liquor on the premises. Some began without this proscription but later found it necessary. One respondent says specifically that most residents in his house have been prescribed tranquilizing drugs and that there are dangers in mixing such drugs and alcohol; whether this is a factor in the decisions of other houses is unknown. Four houses prohibit only "excessive" drinking: "Social drinking is approved when it can be done moderately;" an additional house dropped its official restriction on drinking but finds that custom is maintained and that drinking is moderate and only occasional. Unlike drinking, smoking in the house is rarely prohibited. Only one house forbids it entirely, though most have specific rules about times and places. Many prohibit smoking in bed, for obvious safety reasons, and others prohibit smoking in sleeping rooms.

General middle-class decorum places restrictions on sexual behavior. But in contrast to alcohol, sex is mentioned specifically in the rules of only three houses. Yet it is very probable that almost all houses restrict visits between men and women. Participants in the 1963 conference on halfway houses agree that sexual relations on the premises were universally proscribed, even where not listed among the oral or written rules of halfway houses. Rules for visiting are sometimes stated, limiting time—"no visits after eleven"—and place—"no visits above the first floor." But, as in general society, the topic seems not to be faced openly, and the problems which arise—and there must be some—are dealt with on an individual basis.

The above rules are common either to American middle-class society or to that particular sector of it which defines boarding house life. Nearly all, if not all, halfway houses abide by these codes. There are, however, other rules peculiar to halfway houses which suggest a transitional "halfway" status between mental hospital and community. This group of rules reveals great differences among halfway houses.

Many respondents mention that they expect residents to obey doctors' orders, particularly about medication. Often residents are expected to share in the work of the house, their duties ranging from maintaining only their own rooms to participating in scheduled chores such as dishwashing and general housecleaning. Rural houses usually require and establish hours for farm and maintenance work. Most houses also require some notification by the resident of his leaving the house and his intended time of return. This may be done casually, through a posted sign-out sheet, with simply meal planning and telephone inquiries in mind; or it may be done more restrictively, requiring specific staff assent, in order to be sure at all times where each resident is and his probable occupation. In some houses each resident has his own key; in others there is a specific time—later on weekends than weekdays—by which residents are expected to return to the house.

Some houses require clearance by staff for overnight visits: "Weekend and overnight privileges are granted after the second month of residency, and after conferring with the Social Worker or Rehabilitation Counselor; residents should not plan to be away from the House for more than two weekends each month." Some have rules for phone calls—in one case allowing use of the phone by staff permission only. A number of houses require attendance at particular meetings with purposes ranging from house business to group therapy.

Specific rules vary, and they range from the relatively impersonal codes of an open setting to the highly personal restrictions of the "total" hospital. Thus, some houses will set standards on personal appearance and cleanliness, and one house mentions a specific prohibition on borrowing and lending money between residents. Some other examples of personal restrictions by different houses are:

> Only cash purchases may be made. Credit or lay-away plans are not permitted. Buying, spending . . . and saving should be planned with the Social Worker or Rehabilitation Counselor on a regular budgeting basis.

> Bathroom doors will remain unlocked and Residents are encouraged to shower or bathe at least three times a week. Showers may be taken between: 7:00 a.m.–11:00 p.m.

> One house has a rule against "excessive dating," but notes that the rule is frequently broken.

Much more typical is the fairly open atmosphere implied in the following statements:

We have emphasized the degree of freedom and relative lack of institutional-like rules. Restrictions and limits are almost entirely imposed spontaneously by the men living in the house as part of living together. The men have an effective form of self-government with regular meetings and officers which takes up among other things the setting of house rules. They have evolved such rules as (a) the TV should be turned down very low after 10 p.m., (b) the housekeeper should be notified if a man intends to miss dinner, and (c) the front door is to be locked at 10:30 p.m. The men are told, however, that no drinking is permitted.

There are unwritten rules such as being on time for meals, not disturbing others with loud noise at late hours, respect of others' personal property, no drinking. We have had very little difficulty . . . Most residents are very considerate of others. No rules are frequently broken.

Enforcement of Rules

Where there are rules, written or unwritten, there is the problem of how to make them stick. The method used throughout by halfway houses is primarily that of social pressure. Most often problems of undesirable behavior are dealt with by simple discussion, sometimes with individuals, sometimes with the general group, as at a house meeting. A number of houses report having no behavior problems which fail to be resolved by discussion.

If discussion with other house members or with staff is ineffective, then as a final recourse the resident can be threatened with the possibility that he will be asked to leave the house. Where the liaison between house and hospital is close, or the stay at the halfway house is clearly considered as a sort of trial run immediately following hospitalization, a return to the hospital may always be an implicit threat. In general, however, enforcement of rules does not seem to pose problems for respondents, although specific rules or specific residents may offer difficulty. There is no indication that enforcement is a major issue, and five houses, three of them long established, mention spontaneously that they do not have much difficulty in maintaining cooperative behavior.

Only three houses specifically mention removal of "privileges" as an enforcement device. One uses both restriction on freedom and requirement of additional house chores, commenting that the former is more effective in correcting difficulties than the latter. Another house restricts residents to the house if they come in intoxicated. One house said only that "privileges" were "restricted" as a disciplinary measure.

Thus, the distance of the halfway house from the hospital model is not invariably great. One still sees such inconsistencies as are implied in encouraging a belief in the dignity of work while simultaneously using work as a punishment. Nevertheless, only a very small minority of halfway houses come at all close to the hospital model.

If we measure halfway houses' approaches to rules against a hospital standard, we find them ranging from "quarter-way" to more than "three-quarter-way" in the nature and extent of their rules and in the formality or informality with which these are presented to the resident. Characteristics of the resident population and presumptions—whether based on evidence or not—about the degree of ambiguity which ex-patients can tolerate probably influence the balance considerably. The use of the hospital term "privileges" suggests that the mode of functioning in some houses is rather close to that of the mental hospital. In general, however, most halfway houses have rules which, formalized or not, are considerably less restrictive than those of hospitals. In the greater number of houses the rules and enforcement procedures resemble those of the middle-class community. Indeed, in many houses the rules are no more, and perhaps even less, restrictive than those of an average boarding house. A description by Landy and Greenblatt (1965) vividly shows how a halfway house in its approach to rules differs from the hospital or boarding house:

> In the preadmission interview with Miss Grant [the Director] the resident is unlikely to find out specifically about rules and, in fact,

no formal rules are posted. Therefore during the initial phase she explores the range of behavior sanctions in the House . . .

> One woman told about cooking her first breakfast. Although no one objected when she prepared two eggs she was nervous and apprehensive. "I thought the way I cooked my eggs and everything I did would be reported to the hospital. I didn't know if I was cooking them right. But they don't make you feel they are watching." She further described how she learned what to do and not to do: "You can't bring guests in to dinnertime: that I know from asking the other girls. But I haven't asked Miss Grant. I wouldn't, perhaps, go and bake a cake. I think maybe they wouldn't want me to, but nothing has been said." Actually, as this resident later discovered, they are encouraged to bake cakes for themselves or for relatives and friends. She also learned that guests are permitted on weekends, when there is room due to leaves.

> Another resident said, "I was concerned about whether, if you can't sleep at night, you can really get up and go downstairs. Nobody seemed to mind; there was no rule. So this morning I couldn't sleep, and I decided to go downstairs and turn the light on. And it was known that I was downstairs but nothing was said" (p. 68).

Landy and Greenblatt comment that these women had recently come from an "open" hospital with a *relatively* (their italics) free and unrestricted atmosphere. Nonetheless, the contrast is great. With regard to enforcement of rules, halfway house personnel are likely to show greater flexibility and greater sensitivity to issues of pathology than is true of either hospital or boarding house:

> . . . Clinical experience suggests that often in the patient's early socialization family rules were inconsistent and contradictory, chaotically administered, rigidly, set at such unrealistically high standards that the individual was incapable of living up to them, and punishments for infractions often disproportionately severe. Therefore rules for living are likely to be a particularly touchy problem for halfway house residents.

> The director is sensitive to this fact and seldom resorts to reprimands even when residents behave in a manner flagrantly opposed to her

own conceptions of what is best and proper for their welfare and safety. For example, one Christmas Eve a male friend of Evelyn's, himself a former patient whom she had met in the hospital, come to take her out. At first she refused to go so he offered to take her and three other residents, two of whom were 16 years old. Because of their youth, a previously unfortunate experience with alcohol by one, and lack of knowledge about the young man's ability to deal effectively with possible contingencies, Miss Grant felt this might be an unhappy arrangement but did not attempt to inflict her opinions. She telephoned Miss Ordway, the hospital social worker, who felt that the caller could manage the situation. The group returned before night curfew, but had been drinking, and one of the 16-year-olds was intoxicated, creating a loud disturbance outside that brought a police cruiser. Mrs. Gorman, on duty then, persuaded the police that she could handle the situation. Miss Grant was faced with the occurrence of the very thing she feared, but did not reprimand or indulge in recriminations.

For some women, in the House as in the hospital, probing into the validity and enforceability of "the way things are supposed to be done" provides an experiment for the resident in learning how far one may go in stretching a point of etiquette and "testing the limits" of behavior. One day Gloria came into the kitchen to talk about a new skirt and hair styles. Her hair was up in pin curls with a net over it. Miss Grant said, "I hope you're not coming to the table like that, Gloria. You had better get it dry before dinner. We don't come to the table looking slipshod." Gloria did not respond but left the room. At dinner she appeared with her hair still in pin curls. Miss Grant said nothing. About halfway through dinner Gloria said, "Miss Grant, look at me, my hair is still up." Miss Grant answered, "I know that perfectly well, Gloria. I don't want to talk about it." The subject was dropped.

Gloria may have had the satisfaction of winning this "round," but probably derived little ultimate satisfaction from such testing of reality limits. In the objective sense, the women "need" Miss Grant and sooner or later most of them seem to make a conscious effort to comply with the few standards she requires. The above incident illustrates again that though the director disapproves of a resident's behavior, she does not insist upon her way, and does not take advantage of the presence of the group further to chastise her. The unity and equanimity of the group take precedence over anything she might wish to do about the provocative behavior of one of its members or the enforcement of "rules" (pp. 68–70).

In general, the handling of rules exemplifies the transitional functions ascribed to halfway houses. Whether rules are written or unwritten seems a relatively minor matter. Because the number of residents in a house is generally small, communication can be direct and simple. Rules and their enforcement can partake of the fluidity, individuality and directness possible in small organizations. The halfway house does not quite represent a family model, but it comes far closer to it than it does to the mental hospital model. Still, the halfway house does not function like a family. In many houses procedures for establishing and enforcing rules are like those of housing cooperatives or fraternities. But again, there are differences, some specific and some general, as in degree of control by authority. There is nothing wholly unique about the way halfway houses handle rules—except for the quality of "inbetweenness."

Chapter 11 WORK

IN ANSWER TO A QUERY ABOUT THE COMPONENTS OF PSYCHOLOGICAL health, Freud spoke of capacities for love and work. Work, however defined, has been up to now a part of man's destiny and a part of his human identity. Its economic and social function has gone without saying. At least up to the present day, man has had to work in order to meet his own needs and maintain a viable society. And perhaps this need in itself has been sufficient to transform historical into personal necessity. It is no surprise that a personal ethic should evolve to make the best of fate and that individual and social demands should collude toward an ethos extolling the private virtues of hard work and the social virtues of production.

Yet there is more to it, for work has a personal meaning within the individual life cycle. Images of skill and competence and their fit as part of a meaningful social order become—either by achievement or lack of it—part of self-image. Nor can play, however involved or demanding of skill, substitute for the image of work. Daniel Bell (1956) suggests that this is so because the notion of play demands a parallel notion of work, that play is a release from the tension of work, and these therefore cannot serve as equivalents for one another. Erikson clarifies the personal meaning of work in a view which is compatible with but more explicit than Bell's. According to Erikson play and work are each psychosocial aspects of successive stages in the human developmental process. The accomplishments or failures at a given developmental stage may contribute to the fate of future stages, but earlier and later stages cannot substitute for one another. One must learn to play before one learns to work, and the images derived from each enter, for better or worse, into later emphases—those of fidelity, love, care, integrity. So it is that lacunae or blights in images of work will burden images of love.

Of work itself, Erikson says: "Ever since his 'expulsion from paradise,' . . . man has been inclined to protest work as drudgery or as slavery, and to consider most fortunate those who seemingly can choose to work or not to work. The fact, however, is that man *must* (italics Erikson's) learn to work, as soon as his intelligence and his capacities are ready to be 'put to work,' so that his ego's power may not atrophy (1964, p. 123)." Opportunities for the development and exercise of a sense of competence are, Erikson believes, essential for psychological growth.

Herein, of course, lies a massive problem. As sociologists and social planners have recognized, changes dating from the industrial revolution have led—for all but a fortunate few—to the progressive meaninglessness of individual work. Increased automation is likely to intensify the problem. What are some of the dimensions of this issue?

One obvious, though perhaps minor factor, has been the increase in physical distance of work from the home, contributing to a psychological distance between work and domestic life. More important is that mass production has required specialization, so that work has become differentiated into multiple, organized part functions. To the individual worker—white or blue collar—only a very small part of the whole is visible. Isolated in repetitive tasks, disconnected from the reality of the final product, the worker has little opportunity for investment in skills or pride of workmanship. Furthermore, technological complexity has resulted in a peculiar polarization: on the one hand, there is the simplification and routinization of work to the point where intrinsic challenges disappear; on the other hand, advanced technology defies the understanding of all but a select, highly trained few. Certainly, menial hard labor, in the usual sense, has decreased. But menial labor, as with the traditional hard work of the farmhand or of the housemaid—whose work according to Luther was no farther from God than that of the priest—was comprehensible. Much present work is not. A Dutch psychiatrist, van den Berg (1961) speaks of the alienation of modern man from his work and he illustrates this with descriptions of the difficulties most of us have in explaining the nature of our work to our children. The comment from the Talmud, "Great is work, for it honors the workman," seems very distant from modern shores.

The compensation is, of course, that conditions of work and reimbursement for work have been wondrously improved: although he has paid a price, man as a worker has increasingly gained both means and time to enjoy the fruits of his labor. If pride in workmanship is gone, it can perhaps be compensated—though not substituted—for by pride in the earning and spending of money. Values become oriented to consumption rather than to work. Whether the new orientation will be tenable and lasting is an issue which American society particularly now confronts.

Work and the Mental Hospital

There is little question that most of those who are so severely disturbed as to be hospitalized have their disturbances reflected in their relation to work. Not only with any severe psychological disability does work suffer. The severely disturbed are preoccupied, in an Eriksonian sense, with issues whose genesis antedates those of workmanship. The absorbing problems they are engaged with are primitive ones of simple trust versus distrust and of self versus non-self; these problems infuse and distort the meaning of work.

Until very recent times, hospitals have given little attention to work programs for inmates. On back wards, particularly, the inmate's life has been characterized by an emptiness exceptional even for total institutions—a kind of crowded solitary confinement where only rising and going to bed, mealtimes, and shifts of personnel mark the rhythm of the days. Work on such wards consists of efforts, spurred by attendants, focussed on ward cleanliness. Typically one sees rounds of patients grudgingly pushing mops and polishing blocks.[1] Often, whether the assumption is that labor is therapeutic or simply that of staff forestalling the devil by making work for idle hands, one sees the same polished floor being polished over and over.

Patients who are more fortunate are set to tasks outside the ward itself. In their specific work details, such jobs may resemble their equivalents in the outside community. But there is no mistaking the difference. Outside one gets paid, and he has some choice of how he spends his earnings. Goffman (1961) comments on this aspect of the interpretative schema of total institutions:

> Since on the outside work is ordinarily done for pay, profit, or prestige, the withdrawal of these motives means a withdrawal of certain interpretations of action and calls for new interpretations. In mental hospitals there are what are officially known as "industrial therapy" and "work therapy"; patients are put to tasks, typically mean ones, such as raking leaves, waiting on tables, working in the laundry, and washing floors. Although the nature of these tasks derives from the working needs of the establishment, the claim presented to the patient is that these tasks will help him to relearn to live in society and that his capacity and willingness to handle them will be taken as diagnostic evidence of improvement (p. 90).

As Goffman adds in a footnote, one should not be too cynical about such "therapies," since such work is considerably more meaningful and pleasant than time on the ward.

Those patients who are knowing enough to "make out" and "work the system" can even accrue an exchange in money or

[1] von Mering and King (1957) discuss these typical hospital routines.

barter. There are often a considerable number of undercover arrangements between staff and patients—carwashing, handyman work, and errand-running—for which payment, although sometimes in the guise of "tipping," is made. Even in hospital jobs where money is not involved, "wise" patients learn that there are extraneous incentives which attach to certain jobs—opportunities for better food, services, interpersonal contacts. In the restricted and stimulus-deprived environment of the hospital, even small incentives become important.

Since the late 1950's mental hospitals have been stimulated by the Office of Vocational Rehabilitation under the impact of amendments to the Vocational Rehabilitation Act of 1954 toward recognition of work activities as a part of hospital programming. Vocational rehabilitation counselors have active roles either within or in collaboration with hospitals. Generally the goals of such recent efforts are conceived of as guidance and training or retraining in vocations. Typically the efforts are instituted just before the patient's discharge to the community; they may carry over after the patient leaves the hospital (Black, 1957, 1959; Black et al., 1960; Brooks, 1960, 1961; Lurie & Pinsky, 1961; Olshansky, 1960). Thus hospital work programs tend to occur at the borderline between the hospital and the community—the ward prior to discharge, the day-hospital, the out-patient services, the sheltered workshop. They are part of transitional and aftercare procedures.

There has been little effort to conceptualize and integrate work within the hospital itself—to make it a meaningful part of life in the hospital and a meaningful part of the psychological milieu of the more seriously disturbed patient. Von Mering and King (1957) discuss a few programs in which work plays a part in the remotivation of so-called chronic patients. Interestingly, such innovative attempts generally start outside the formal channels of the hospital structure. The Cummings recognize the problem of integrating work into the hospital milieu (Cumming & Cumming, 1962). They speak of the importance of work in relation to self-esteem, and they recognize that work involves not only instrumental competence in relation to a task but also group membership and relations with others. In contrast to the usual emphasis on the "better" patient, they suggest that: "For chronic patients who have been desocialized by long stays in a hospital, and for newly admitted patients with long histories of occupational inadequacy, it [work] is the treatment of choice (p. 233–234)." They suggest the creation of artificial work groups of no more than twelve patients, where simple activities are encouraged: "It does not matter too much what [the patients] do so long as they do something with meaning (p. 237)."

A program such as this may be extremely valuable in achieving the aims emphasized by the Cummings: maximizing aspects of group living and opportunities for social interaction and communication. A similar program is described by Appleby *et al.* (1960); but Appleby *et al.* distinguish such activity programs from work. Landy and Raulet (1959) attempt finer differentiations: recreational therapy, ". . . activity which may be classed as entertainment, but in which nothing actually may be produced;" occupational therapy, ". . . in which something is produced which is primarily of value to [the patient];" and industrial work therapy, in which "energies are expended toward accomplishment of something of use to others (p. 74)." They further note the limits on the range and variety of tasks available in the hospital setting and the strains which tend to engender the use of work as punishment. One may question whether the psychological functions of work can be fulfilled without including elements of choice, social usefulness, and remuneration. Rational planning for hospital patients thus is confounded by failure to distinguish between programs of actual work and programs designed to inculcate a psychological base for work attitudes.

The Halfway House and Work

Since halfway houses are for the most part committed to bringing the resident into a closer integration with the general community, it is reasonable to expect that they will concern themselves with the employment of their residents. For the formerly disabled ex-mental patient, work can provide: (a) a source of income; (b) the satisfaction that some form of productivity gives; (c) a measure of respect for himself and for others; and, (d) a socialized way of occupying time. Some halfway houses, as we have noted, use potential employability as a basis for selecting residents. Yet most patients leaving hospitals do not have immediate prospects of getting and holding jobs, and even those who at one time had marketable skills are likely to have lost them if their period of hospitalization or inactivity has been long.

Some houses leave all job concerns to the resident himself; others play an extremely active role in moving the resident toward work. Most provide some direction. If the first attempt of a halfway house is to stir a resident into some kind of activity, the next is to try to get him into a work or work-like situation. This can happen very naturally in a rural farm setting where chores are essential and are continuously renewing themselves. On a farm there is no need for "made" work, and although opportunities for paid jobs may be few, men as well as women can fulfill traditional roles. An urban house does not have as many necessary maintenance duties, and jobs in an urban community often seem less easily adaptable to individual incapacities. Consequently, for the resident newly released from a mental hospital, urban halfway houses must often rely on volunteer work or rehabilitation centers (where they exist) to accustom the resident to the requirements of the working situation before he is ready to attempt a regular job.[2]

With a few exceptions—for instance, with rural houses where farm and maintenance work are needed on the premises, or where there are administrative reasons, as with one Veterans Administration house which, because it was still part of a hospital, had to restrict residents from receiving pay—almost all houses

[2] The possibilities of close and effective working relations among mental hospital, vocational rehabilitation services, and halfway house are illustrated in Brooks' discussion of the Vermont houses (1959).

encourage residents to get paying jobs. In 80% of the houses surveyed some residents worked either part or full time at gainful employment outside of the house. At only six of the forty houses was no one working at an outside job.

Although almost all houses encourage work and in the greater proportion of houses *some* residents do have jobs, there remains the question of how many residents achieve gainful employment. The questionnaire asked about numbers of residents holding paying jobs. The data appear in Table 7, which summarizes approximate percentages of residents employed in each house. Excluding inapplicable replies, the median percentage of employed would seem to fall between 26 and 45%; no house had more than 65% of its residents in paying jobs. Thus, although there are employed residents living in most houses, only a relatively small proportion of residents seem to be involved in paid employment. Unfortunately the question about number of employed residents, although legitimate at face value is too equivocal to yield other than tentative leads. The percentages may indicate that many residents are, despite encouragement, unable either to find or to hold jobs—a not unexpected possibility since a considerable number have come to the halfway house after long periods of hospitalization. On the other hand, the low percentages may relate to admission and turnover policies. Unless a house makes paid employment a contingency for admitting a new resident— and no house to our knowledge does that—it is likely that there will be a period in which new residents do not have jobs; percentages will thus vary with proportions of new to old residents. Employment will also, of course, depend on prevailing economic conditions.

An alternative approach would be to ask about numbers of residents gainfully employed at the end of their stay in the house—a question which moves into the area of evaluating halfway house performance. Although there are no definitive data, two reports are suggestive. In sampling a year's operation, Conard House reports that in its population of 40 residents, 24 were considered successful on the basis of sustained employment without intervening hospitalization; 5 residents returned to the hospital; and 11 others moved to the larger community but lacked employment (Conard House, 1963). Woodley House in an Annual Report for 1965 indicates that 26 out of their 44 residents during the year were in full-time paid work by the end of their stay; 7 attended school; 4 took part in day-hospital programs; 2 did volunteer work; and 5 were without regular occupation.

Most often, according to the questionnaire data, residents find jobs on their own. In other cases rehabilitation counselors and rehabilitation services take the major role in getting employment for the resident. Less usual sources for jobs are public and private employment agencies, friends and relatives, houseparents, other residents and ex-residents. Responses to the questionnaire suggest that finding a job for the resident requires strong motivation on the part of someone. That someone may be the resident himself; alternatively it may be a vocational counselor, the house manager, or a person who is interested in helping ex-patients or the particular halfway house.

TABLE 7. Approximate Percentage of Residents Holding Outside Paying Jobs

	Number of Houses
No employed residents	6
25% or less employed	11
26 to 45% employed	10
46 to 65% employed	9
Over 65% employed	0
Some employed but number not given	2
Question not answered	2
	40

The questionnaire does not tell of the intensity of efforts expended in securing employment for residents. The fact that at least a quarter of the houses are actively involved in state or national vocational rehabilitation programs suggests, in itself, that the matter of employment is given considerable emphasis. Informal discussion strengthens this impression; as one might expect, the ability of the resident to hold a self-sustaining job is seen as one major, if not *the* major, criterion of the halfway house's success in integrating the resident to the broader social community.

Despite such emphasis, there is considerable variation in how active or passive a role a house plays. Almost all houses exert general social pressures on their residents. But some go beyond this by building into their structures special forms of encouragement; others, despite seeming encouragement of employment, have structural arrangements which subvert it.

One form of encouragement is by special concessions made for those working in outside jobs. Of the 32 houses having employed residents, ten say that they make some such concessions. These generally consist of special arrangements for meals or other minor changes to suit the convenience of working residents; three houses, furthermore, lighten the household chores of those having jobs. In contrast, there are two houses which require higher payment for board and room of those residents with outside employment, the rationale being that the employed resident performs less work about the house. Thus, whatever their explicit policies may be, these houses in effect penalize the resident who holds a job.

There are other forms of encouragement toward employment. For example, Woodley House has an ingenious incentive system which provides a clear and constant reminder of the importance of finding a socially-valued occupation outside the house. Productive activity—defined as that which helps either the resident or the community namely, study, volunteer work, or regular employment—is encouraged by the rate structure. Residents who remain at home must pay a far higher fee than those who get out into some productive activity. One may rationalize this scheme by the fact that the resident spending less time at the house requires less staff attention. The incentive plan may backfire—as with a resident who, intent on punishing her parents who paid her fees, deliberately refused work—but it rarely does. There is yet another way in which Woodley House encourages work. Social activity at the house during the day could conceivably lower the impetus of the resident to seek a job outside the house. Woodley House therefore intentionally maintains an uneventful daytime atmosphere at the house so that a resident is less likely to feel much conflict about leaving the house in the morning.

Other houses are active in establishing relations and fostering contact with possible employers. The potential intensity of such programs for assisting the resident to break into the working world is best illustrated by the ingenious and carefully worked out plans of Fountain House (Goertzel, Beard, & Pilnick, 1960; Beard *et al.*, 1964). Fountain House, in New York City, obtained the cooperation of a number of local industries, which allotted a number of jobs to the program. The jobs and the working environment are pre-tested by Fountain House staff—generally social workers —so as to determine the amount and kinds of stress peculiar to each job. The positions are then held successively by Fountain House ex-patient members.

A group of employers in New York City agreed to give to Fountain House one or more of their job positions, which [Fountain House] could use for purely rehabilitative purposes. These jobs, paying regular rates, ranged from clerical work in a large Fifth Avenue store to messenger work in a small printing company. A Fountain House member is permitted to work on a job placement for as little as one hour per day, if necessary.

Each job is performed first by a social worker in order to determine the performance standards which the member, when placed, must meet in order to achieve a successful job experience. Also, the worker is able to identify those tensions unique to the job environment. By working on each new job placement, the professional worker is also able to secure the interest and cooperation of fellow employees. He can explain and interpret the rehabilitative function of the job placement which is to be initiated.

Each job placement is limited to three or four months. Hours of work are gradually increased as the member's tolerance for work and self-confidence increases. Of course, the worker can always accompany the patient at any time during the job placement. This is found to be particularly helpful when the member is experiencing difficulties on the job. After a member has demonstrated to himself and to his employer his capacity to perform work, he then moves on to a job of his own, the placement being used over again by another member (Beard *et al.*, 1964, pp. 17–18).

Other houses use other means in helping residents prepare themselves for getting and holding jobs. Among these means are: (*a*) vocational rehabilitation counseling at the house; (*b*) staff help in writing job application forms; (*c*) role-playing sessions with staff and peers to give the resident practice and confidence in undertaking job interviews.[3] Failures of ex-patients in finding and maintaining employment are likely to derive at least as much from interpersonal problems as from work-skill problems. And it is in the more personal aspects that halfway houses can be most helpful.

The major incentive to work no doubt remains money and its significance for satisfying both practical and social wishes. In contrast to the hospital, most halfway houses positively sanction earning of money. In 21 of the 32 houses which have working residents, the use of income from work is at the sole discretion of the resident himself; at other houses, residents are encouraged to share responsibility with staff by discussing their expenditures; at only one house—where the population consists of adolescents— does the management take principal charge of the resident's in-

[3] One common issue which all ex-patients face is whether or not to tell prospective employers of their hospitalization. Some houses recommend that employers be informed, while others consider the matter one which the individual resident must work out entirely for himself. Others suggest that the information be communicated only if it has some particular pertinence. In telling an employer of a previous hospitalization, an applicant may be unconsciously asking for special consideration while overtly declaring his desire to be treated exactly like any other employee. By refraining from giving this information where refraining is possible and reasonable, the job seeker simplifies the situation for his employer and assures that he will be judged on his working record alone. This does not, of course, solve the problem of how an applicant can account for the time he has spent out of employment when that is a requirement of application. See Olshansky (1959) for a discussion of the general problem of employer receptivity.

come. Money from sources other than work, can, of course, act as a negative incentive. Participants at the 1963 Woodley House Conference reported least success in achieving employment among residents who had benefits or pensions which would be lost as a result of earning money. Obviously, threat of loss of welfare or pension support is not always a determining factor, but any reduction in motivation can act to reduce the likelihood of jobs being sought, or that, if found, they will work out satisfactorily. In Fountain House's very active transitional employment program, arrangements are made so that members supported by welfare or other funds experience a net gain in income through work (Beard, Schmidt, & Smith, 1963).

Volunteer Work

Volunteer work may not have all the values of paid work. Still, it preserves many of them, and it may be used as a trial-run for those still unable to compete successfully in the job market. Many of the requirements of volunteer work are similar to those of paid work. One must meet schedules of time and place, and one must carry through the specific tasks of a job. Volunteer work can provide a sense of personal accomplishment and social usefulness; it can help the resident understand or remember the requirements of working. At the same time it may have the advantage of being less demanding than full-time paid employment. Unfortunately, it does not reward the worker with a paycheck at the end of the week, nor does it give him full confidence that he has passed the test of real work. Limited volunteer efforts may be less tension-producing than full-time paid employment, but they may also be less gratifying. Nevertheless, such work—partly because of its voluntary nature—carries more dignity and meaning than do usual patient hospital tasks. Its special character makes it a suitable stepping stone toward fuller vocational efforts. Of the 40 houses in the survey, 19 said that their residents held volunteer jobs sometimes; 15 said they did not; and 6 did not answer the question.

Work in the House

In the questionnaire section on *Work and Jobs*, it was asked whether the residents contributed work which would otherwise require staff or hired labor. One respondent failed to answer the item. Fifteen houses said that care of the resident's own room was all that was expected. Twenty-four of the 40 houses did expect extra labor beyond care of the rooms. Of these, seven said that tasks were either formally assigned to residents or combined both formal assignment and the resident's own initiative; in the remaining seventeen houses the extra work was undertaken by the resident only by his own choosing. Just how large a part the efforts of residents play in the totality of necessary work around the house presumably differs from halfway house to halfway house, just as it does from one ordinary household to another. Where there are a large number of residents and only houseparents or only a housemother and occasional help, clearly a considerable responsibility falls to the residents. Nevertheless, despite differences among houses, there is an overwhelming similarity. In contrast to the hospital, the arrangements for work within the house seem predominantly based on an ethic of sharing in common tasks; work distribution is for the most part informal and homelike.

Summary

Halfway houses in general devote considerable effort to the matter of work and jobs for their residents. Within these general efforts is considerable variation in the specifics of design and in the degree of activity and support provided by staff. In no case, however, is there any impression of "made work," such as the aimless floor mopping characteristic of many hospitals, nor is there evidence of any emphasis on considering as work typical hospital craft activities which may serve expressive functions but have little or no social value in the world beyond the hospital. For the halfway house, in sharp contrast to the hospital, work—

whether paid, volunteer, or within the house—is real work. Yet the degree of support and encouragement and the professional efforts devoted to introducing the resident to this real work is far greater than that not only of boarding houses but also of other agencies such as out-patient and welfare clinics. The transitional function of a halfway house is perhaps seen most clearly in its mediation of the work status of the residents.

We have in this chapter addressed ourselves primarily to issues concerning the individual resident in his adjustment to work. But questions about the potentialities of halfway houses for mediating the work status of its residents go beyond purely individual concerns. Patients in hospitals are a high cost to the community. Those released from hospitals to live on welfare funds continue to drain community resources. In contrast, Beard, Schmidt, and Smith (1963) note that the 25 members who graduated from the Fountain House placement project and who held jobs in 1963 earned a total of $75,000 a year. Many of these had previously required support through welfare or family funds. In another report (Beard, Pitt, Fisher, & Goertzel, 1963), Fountain House notes the superior employment record of those undertaking its program in contrast to a well-selected control group. When one considers average life spans and long term losses and gains, intensive efforts toward improving the employability of the mentally disturbed pay off, not only in essential human terms, but also in the economics of the broader community.

Chapter 12　THERAPY

THERE IS NOTHING PERMANENT EXCEPT CHANGE, SAID HERACLITUS. For the fact of change, no special theory is needed. Given a world in which our knowledge of future events is probabilistic rather than certain, and given some measure of uncertainty in the contingencies of response to an imperfectly predictable environment, change is inevitable. The wonder is rather that we are able to draw some constancies out of the ever-changing flux.

Of the conditions and circumstances for change, we know something, but what we know is far short of enabling us to predict or plan the course of human affairs with total assurance. We can perhaps say something about which contingencies among events will tend toward a particular set of outcomes. This we do, not only in such broad areas as economic and social planning, but also in each moment of our daily lives. Our actions and conversations, our schedules and plans presume trends. But outcomes are seldom quite certain. Not only are there unforeseen circumstances—the accidents by which actions go askew and plans awry—but there are also the possibilities of systematic changes which will steer a course of events into new directions.

It is with these possibilities of systematic change that we are here concerned. The questions we face are how one establishes and maintains change in new directions. Under ordinary circumstances we have some proximate answers to these questions. When we are growing up, for example, the world we live in often points the way. When we are children our parents, as representatives of that world, reinforce our choice of some directions rather than others, and we in turn socialize our children according to the views we have of the world. But simple reinforcement is only one of the devices by which our directions change. Development, both physical and intellectual, also presses us to new modes of conception and new patterns of behavior. Given proper conditions, our thoughts, actions, feelings and fantasies shift with the phases of our life cycle so as to reflect systematic change while maintaining personal continuity. Moreover, and again if circumstances are favorable, we seek conditions under which new learning can occur. Curiosity and exploration, though they may become inhibited, seem built-in not only for humans but also for other far lower mammalian species. We seek information and even at times profit from it prior to any reinforcement, changing our patterns of behavior and moving into new patterns which expand our physical and psychological worlds. The forces of environmental reinforcement, of developmental change, and of exploration and mastery all contribute to the emergence of new adaptive patterns.

The qualification, "if circumstances are favorable," appears in all the above comments. Specific learning, developmental growth and adaptation, exploration and information seeking are normative processes. It is when these normative processes are inhibited or fail that we are faced with the questions of psychological pathology: what are the conditions of failure and what are the conditions for reinstating normal functioning?

We need first of all to recognize that deviance in itself does not necessarily imply a disturbance in normative processes. For example, the visitor from a foreign culture may behave inappropriately by our standards because he has not learned these standards. Similarly, subcultural differences, as between socioeconomic classes, produce discrepancies whereby what is normal to one group appears deviant to another. In the past mental health workers have been too prone to view what differed from their own social and value standards as indicative of personal pathology, and only recently, through the influence of sociological studies, have they begun to realize that socially disturbing deviance, such as gang delinquency, does not necessarily reflect personal psychological disturbance. Where normative processes are intact, the creation of change, in directions deemed favorable, requires providing appropriate opportunities for learning, for maturation and development, and for seeking and gaining information.

To provide such opportunities is by no means an easy task. To influence socialization, so that it goes in one direction rather than another according to plan, requires both theoretical knowledge and practical control. We are short on both sides. Our knowledge of normative processes of function, our knowledge of environments and of modes of changing and optimizing environments is limited; our power to manipulate and change the world according to our psychological orientations is also limited. And beyond these limitations lie perplexing and critical questions of social and ethical philosophies.

It is one thing to attempt to institute change under the assumption that a system is intact but has somehow gotten off on a wrong track. It is another matter when the system itself seems to have broken down. In cases of severe psychopathology—as in the schizophrenias, which constitute by far the greatest diagnostic bulk of mental hospital patients—we seem to be faced with such a breakdown. Learning is primitivized; developmental change is inhibited; exploration and information seeking and utilization are sharply restricted.[1]

If, in severe disturbance, we are dealing with a breakdown in normative processes, then we can hardly depend much on these processes in our attempts to institute change. The tasks of socialization or re-socialization require some degree of sensitivity to the world on the part of the subject. Certainly even the most severely disturbed retain a sufficient capacity for recognizing punishment

[1] Although life in a mental hospital may, as we have suggested, foster the delimitations which come with breakdown, it does not in itself produce them.

and reward so that immediate and localized ward behavior can be changed (Ayllon & Haughton, 1962; Ayllon & Michael, 1959), and it is important to note that even at this level of primitivization dramatic alterations of ward behavior are possible through manipulation of environmental contingencies. Still the laboriousness of such steps suggests that we are not dealing with normal, though misdirected, processes. The problem remains one, not of altering behavior, but of establishing or re-establishing the ordinary human sensibilities necessary to respond to and profit from the circumstances of the world.

To change the environment may be of rather limited use to one who no longer lives in the world. If the schizophrenic has "cut out of it," giving up human capacities and abnegating human status, to be brought into the world means more than simply reacting to new contingencies so as to avoid punishment or so as to get the reward of a piece of candy. It means developing some minimum sense of trust and hope in oneself and one's fellow man, a confidence that there is sufficient order in the world and in oneself so that one can try to make these meet. Those who have been successful in changing the long-term chronic schizophrenic and in changing not simply deviant behavior, but rather the person who chooses to behave as a deviate, have all had to meet the subject in his world before imposing their own worlds upon him (Fromm-Reichmann, Knight, Rosen, Sechehaye, Sullivan, Will).[2] They have had to establish some understanding of the world of the disturbed as a foundation for a relation of trust. They have had to rely on this relation sufficiently so that it in turn could become a base for the institution, or reinstitution, of learning, development, and information seeking and utilization.

Other approaches seek some substitute for the intensive, long-term, emotionally demanding—and also expensive and time-consuming—work that is psychotherapy with the schizophrenic,

---

[2] Cf. Fromm-Reichmann, 1950; Knight, 1946; Rosen, 1953; Sechehaye, 1951; Sullivan, 1953; Will, 1961. An illuminating account of the personal struggles one encounters in intensive work with schizophrenics is presented by Farber (1966a, 1966b).

while they maintain the orientation of psychotherapy: that what is at issue is not behavior, per se, but rather a sense of personal worth, of hope, of faith in other humans. Such approaches may focus on any of a wide variety of areas—including such emphases as accomplishments in work, environmental supports, or improvements in family communications. The specific foci may be very different from that of the individual psychotherapy relationship; but, as in psychotherapy, concern is not totally nor primarily with behavioral symptoms. Rather, in such approaches, disturbed and disturbing behavior are viewed as manifestations of more fundamental problems. And the particular approach is dictated by its theory about the fundamental problem.

What are the fundamental problems of severe disturbance? Once more, we must here remind ourselves of our ignorance. Are we dealing with disease? The notion of disease requires some notion of specific etiology. The causes of schizophrenia have been argued as genetic, as metabolic, as neurologic, as psychogenic, as social—with all sorts of variations within and between these. There is no conclusive, incontrovertible evidence for any of these positions. If schizophrenia is a disease, its ranges of symptoms and its courses of development are remarkably varied. There have been arguments that the phenomena of schizophrenia represent the manifestations of not one but a variety of diseases. On the other hand, recent discussions suggest that schizophrenia represents a degree of psychological disorganization that is part of a single continuum of all mental illness (Menninger, 1960; Menninger et al., 1958). Again, we may note here our earlier discussion in Chapter 2, and Szasz's critique of the entire concept of mental disorder as disease.

If there is no agreement on the nature of schizophrenia as a disease, or indeed on whether it is many diseases or none at all, there are as many differences of opinion with respect to notions of treatment. Physical treatments of various kinds have been espoused, from surgical procedures through shock to drugs, sometimes on a basis of elaborate theories of brain function, sometimes with no theory at all. Environmental treatments have ranged from foci on specific aspects of ward procedures to programs involving inter-relations between hospital and the broader community. More directly personal approaches have ranged from educative efforts directed at socialization through a variety of integrative efforts directed at the individual, or his group, or his family. Moreover, all sorts of combinations among physical, environmental, and personal treatments continue to be tried.

It might seem that research could easily clarify some of these issues, that it could tell us which of these approaches work and which do not. But the problems are not that simple. Each approach has its successes—patients improve in their behavior on hospital wards and discharge rates increase—at least for a while. Are such results, as some have argued, simply a "Hawthorne effect"—a thesis, named after a series of industrial studies, that any procedure, so long as it provides an indication of attention and interest, improves the work performance of employees? Or is it that each approach influences a different sub-population of the hospitalized? How does one avoid investigator biases, and what sort of control studies are necessary? And there is another question, which we shall consider later: Is an investigatory model based on a paradigm of illness and treatment appropriate for the study of psychological disturbance and its modification?

Therapy and the Halfway House

It is no wonder then that the term "therapy" has such multiple and diverse meanings, many of which are vague and confusing. And in retrospect it is no wonder that the questionnaire items on *Therapy* (Appendix A, Item 46a to 46i), although they seemed reasonable enough on the surface, left something wanting in terms of replies. For example, at almost all houses tranquilizing drugs were prescribed for some residents. Obviously, some respondents regarded their use as therapy. Such diverse programs as vocational training, milieu modifications, recreational activities, drug prescriptions, meetings with groups or individuals (whether or not under a formal designation as therapy), and even the encouragement of pleasant social interactions, all may turn out to be someone's notion of "therapy."[3] The questionnaire items were probably neither sufficiently specific nor unambiguous enough to enable unequivocably clear interpretation.

Nonetheless, the halfway house is an institution committed to change. What sets it apart from other nonhospital residential environments is not simply that it accepts ex-patients as residents. In its commitment to helping the patient make the transition from separation to integration within the general community, the halfway house undertakes to foster development and change in this direction. At each of the houses, whether or not they use the word "therapy" to describe it, there is a conscious attempt to provide an atmosphere and set of circumstances conducive to helping a troubled person feel capable and interested enough to renew his activities in the world.

Only four houses of the sample of forty state that they have no program of therapy (Table 8), but in view of the considerations noted above, the figure is difficult to interpret. For example, one house, which specifically disclaims providing any therapy, says it exists "to meet some of the needs . . . of people [for] acceptance, love, fellowship . . . to effect their restoration of confidence and reorientation to life and hope;" its respondent adds that pastoral counseling is the "only form of so-called therapy" offered. Another house, similar in its spiritual and religious orientation, also disclaims therapy and counts on healthy living in a benevolent atmosphere to effect favorable changes in their residents. Such houses, apart from their lack of medical directorship, seem close spiritual descendents of the enlightened early and mid-nineteenth century era of "moral treatment."

Confusion about the word "therapy," and rejection of the notion that activities within the house should be considered as or directed toward therapy are, however, by no means a sign of lack of psychological sophistication. In fact it is the more active, sophisticated halfway houses which raise such questions. One house, for

[3] One respondent referring to house activities says, "There is no end to group therapy in this situation;" others mention good food, trips, cultural activities, tutoring, and "book work."

example, although it specifically rejects the rubric of therapy for its within-house activities, has a staff which is highly sensitive and knowledgeable in dealing with the personal pathologies and strengths of its residents, and seeks, through consultation, to maximize its effectiveness in working with residents. Another house, all of whose residents are in treatment with individual therapists outside the house, consciously deemphasizes any "therapeutic" orientation which would tend to give the house the atmosphere of a hospital or convalescent home, rather than that of a community. A third house which does not build any systematic group or individual psychotherapy into its program states that its "therapy consists primarily of regular association with nonpatients, nonpatient values and expectations and the requirements that individuals perform in productive social roles." That this statement represents far more than a token, offhand remark is suggested by the respondent's further comments:

> We have tried to operationalize these conceptions: (1) In the interest of resocialization, as soon as possible the patient should relinquish all attributes of the patient status, i.e., he is not referred to as "patient," he is "expected" to be able to enjoy full-citizen status— he comes and goes with freedom, he performs on an equal basis with others, etc. (2) An ex-patient should be a part of a group which resembles structures found in the larger society—not ones associated with life inside a hospital; thus the house mixes patients and nonpatients, males and females, etc. (3) The institution for rehabilitating or resocializing should vary with the type of population served. For some, the chronic patient, for example, the institution of "family" is considered more appropriate than that of professionally organized treatment based on the model of individual psychotherapy or group psychotherapy. Thus, "treatment" consists in the manipulation of structures in the social system in which the ex-patient has membership—e.g., the role system is expanded or changed, special operating norms are introduced specifically for their resocialization value, etc.

In this chapter we consider primarily the issues of halfway houses in relation to formal psychotherapy and secondarily some problems of drug treatment. Approaches to change which focus on the social milieu are considered in the following chapter.

Psychotherapy

Despite divergent views about what is and what is not therapy, it was apparent that most respondents answered the questionnaire items as though these referred to psychotherapy. The tone was probably set by the items themselves, but this direction was no doubt also partly determined by current orientations in the field.

Where and By Whom

At most houses, formal programs of therapy—that is, efforts apart from work with the house milieu—are separated from house activities. Therapy programs take place outside the house in 25 of the 40 cases (Table 8). This is true for all 13 houses affiliated with the Veterans Administration. Their residents generally enter the halfway house for a trial visit before formal discharge from the hospital. Throughout their stay at the halfway house these residents may continue to be seen by psychotherapists or caseworkers who are affiliated with the hospital. The situation often provides continuity in the transition between hospital and halfway house, since a resident can continue with the same therapist. In some cases those serving as therapists in both the VA hospital and its affiliated halfway house also function as consultants to the house director.

In twelve non-VA houses all formally constituted therapy took place outside the house. Here the design varies somewhat from the VA model. In six of these houses the pattern is very close to that of the VA houses in their having close working associations with hospitals and continuing therapy for their ex-patients with therapists at the hospitals. A difference from the VA pattern is that more than a single hospital may be involved. Two additional houses have similar arrangements, except that the association is with outpatients clinics rather than with hospitals. The remaining four houses use a variety of resources, including private practitioners, as agents for outside therapy.

When therapy is described as occurring outside the house, it almost always means either individual or group psychotherapy, and in by far the most cases individual therapy. The meaning is more ambiguous for the ten of the forty houses where therapy is described as taking place within the house. For example, at one house the director called it "tutoring" and presumably conducted it as such. At another there was a carefully considered milieu program and an emphasis on the relationship between normal college student residents and ex-patients. At one rural house an actively planned work program, as well as group and individual therapy, provided a range of therapeutic effort. Recreational and vocational training were mentioned by two houses. Some four houses, where therapy was said to take place within the house, appeared to concentrate on group therapy and group vocational counseling.

TABLE 8.   Where Therapy Takes Place

	Number of Houses
Inside the house	10
Outside the house:	
VA	13
Non-VA	12
Both inside and outside the house	1
No therapy program	4
	40

In the 25 cases in which formal therapy was outside of the house, respondents were asked whether being in therapy was set as a condition of residence. In only nine cases was an active relation with a therapist mandatory. In the mandatory non-VA cases the individual therapist was often the primary referral source, and a continuing relationship was maintained between house and therapist. Although the remaining 16 of these 25 houses did not make therapy a condition of residence, they all appeared to encourage it.

As in other parts of the survey, there is a considerable diversity, this time in the disciplines represented among therapists. Most frequently mentioned, with nineteen references, are psychi-

atrists; then come social workers with seventeen; and psychologists
with fourteen.[4] There are a very few references to non-psychiatric
physicians, occupational therapists and recreational workers and not
many to vocational counselors probably because their roles were
more often thought of by respondents in connection with the questionnaire section on *Work and Jobs.*

Respondents were also asked about schedules for consultation with therapists: whether such consultations occurred formally
and at regular intervals or informally according to need. Only one
house definitely had no consultation, although seven found the
item inapplicable, perhaps because therapy was occurring solely
with house staff. Thus eighty percent of the houses ($N=32$) maintained a program of consultation. Consultation was usually informal
($N=20$), but eleven houses had formally scheduled conferences
at regular intervals or combinations of formal and informal consultations. These data are presented in Table 9.

TABLE 9. Consultation with Therapists

Consultation	N
Formal and at regular intervals	4
Informal according to need	20
Both formal and informal	7
Does not say	1
No Consultation	
No consultation	1
No answer	7
	40

Problems of Therapy

The respondents were asked about problems in relation to
their programs for therapy. Among the ten houses whose conception it was to have therapy take place within the house, there was

---

[4] The frequencies added to more than forty, since most often more than
one discipline was mentioned.

considerable feeling of need for improvement. The comments, however, reflect only local issues—the need for better recreational facilities, or certain physical improvements, or a group therapy program—and offer no generalizations. The replies of the remaining respondents indicate that special problems do arise when therapy takes place outside the halfway house. There are indications of occasional disagreements with psychotherapists over the behavior of individual residents. A therapist may, for example, feel that the house should be more tolerant than it is of his patient's deviance; the position of the halfway house is often that it cannot always focus on what might be best for a particular resident, since it must consider the effects of its policies and actions in relation to all its residents. The individual, prescriptive orientation of the personal therapist may conflict with the emphasis of the house on processes of group living. To house staff, the therapist's proposals regarding his client may suggest a catering to psychopathology. To the therapist, the house's efforts to orient the resident toward the community may seem premature and harsh. Added to these are often problems of high turnover among therapists at hospitals and clinics, problems seen by some respondents as complicating and as lowering the effectiveness of their houses' therapy programs. It is no wonder then that a relatively frequent comment on sources of difficulty has to do with communication problems between therapists and the halfway house staff.

Yet there are clear advantages in keeping anything resembling formal psychotherapy *outside* the house, as do about 70 percent of the houses which claim to have therapy programs. Some reasons are hinted at by two houses which had and abandoned group psychotherapy programs in the house itself. If the psychotherapist is also a staff person, there is confusion between the requirements of these two roles. For the resident there is also confusion—between being a house member and being a patient. One house, whose residents are all in psychotherapy with outside therapists, comments specifically on its efforts to avoid within the house the special institutional atmosphere associated with therapy, clinics, or hospitals. Another house comments on its policies of not duplicating the functions of other institutions and of encouraging the resident "to seek outside help—socially or therapeutically—just as he will need to do when he leaves the house." Psychotherapists are one community resource among others and it is logical for halfway houses to maintain that—in contrast to the situation in "total institutions"—such resources be sought in the community.

Having outside persons as therapists does not dispose of all problems which need to be solved. The therapist is often the referring source of the resident to the house. His continued relationship with the resident is one of influence and indeed power. Conflicts between psychotherapist and halfway house tend to be fought out with the resident as battleground and to his detriment. Attempting to forestall and alleviate such difficulties, participants at the Woodley House Conference (1963) arrived at the following recommendations:

1. Before the resident moves in there should be a clear understanding between the therapist and the staff and the therapist may be called upon for help and consultation at any time should the resident become especially upset.

2. The therapist and the house staff should keep one another informed, by agreed-upon means (either formal or informal conferences or correspondence), of any significant changes in the resident or his situation.

3. It is desirable for the therapists to have visited the house and to have come to an understanding of the conditions generally prevailing in the house. Such a visit may help the therapist determine more accurately whether the house situation is likely to be a beneficial one for his patient; it also provides a solid basis for communication with the house staff.

Drugs

Although the questionnaire section on *Therapy* included parenthetically the mention of chemotherapy, there was no follow-up of questions relating to medication. Some respondents did mention drugs; that others did not is no indication of whether or not residents were under medication. Informal comments among participants at the Woodley House Conference suggest that a very large proportion of halfway house residents use tranquilizing drugs to some extent. Since such drugs may be powerful, there is serious concern about possible misuse, and a special problem of halfway houses is in the management of drugs. A resident might take too many or too few. Medication may be left carelessly about and come to be used by someone other than the person for whom it was intended.

Each halfway house has its own particular method of handling the problem of drugs. Some houses give all control of drugs to the resident. Some dole them out in much the same fashion as do hospitals. Some use the graduation to personal responsibility for drug-taking as a reward for, or a recognition of, the resident's increasing acceptance of responsibility. Some houses give out only a few days' supply of drugs at a time; others store drugs in a central location readily accessible to residents, but where their use can be observed and private supplies cannot be accumulated. Halfway house directors seem agreed that no system of drug management can be truly foolproof—that every house works out a system of its own, but that all systems incur a certain amount of risk. Though minimized, such risks also exist in hospitals. The best preventive measure is the alertness of administrators to the possible misuse of drugs by those with access to them; this awareness should aid in preventing actual misuse.

One Woodley House Conference participant noted that a special obligation of the house administrative staff is to inform the physician when drug therapy seems out of balance or ineffective for a resident. The physician, who must prescribe on the basis of little personal knowledge of the resident, cannot possibly have the same total awareness of the resident's reactions as does the house staff who spend so much more time with him. A sharing of this knowledge with the physician may be most important in helping him to prescribe effectively and thus facilitate significantly the resident's readjustment to community life.

Chapter 13   THE SOCIAL ENVIRONMENT

THE HALFWAY HOUSE GREW OUT OF FORCES FOR CHANGE. AS DIS-
cussed in Chapter 2, and indeed throughout this book, its design
arose as a possible answer to questions raised about the operations
of the traditional mental hospital. The more conservative houses
question only a few aspects of the hospital; the more radically innovative reject the hospital model in its entirety. For some it is
simply that some aspects of hospital style are inappropriate for
those who are at the edge of return to the community; for others
it is simply that hospitals are bad places for people whatever their
psychological state.

Certainly, halfway houses differ from hospitals in each of
the aspects we have so far examined: their ecological setting, size
and architecture; their approaches to rules, to work, to therapy;
the terms they use—*living rooms* rather than *day-rooms, residents,
clients* or *guests* rather than *inmates* or *patients.* Massive structural
differences are implied in the two words "house" and "hospital."[1]

---

[1] The structural differences relate, in part, to differences in goals. The
mental hospital has been forced into a custodial role. Smith (1965) notes that
the logic of custody creates inherent contradictions which make the welfare of the
individual inmate precarious. The custodial role imposed by the community
upon the hospital tends to make "playing it safe" the guiding principle above
all others, and this, Smith suggests, favors coercion and reduced autonomy for
the individual patient.

And out of the structural differences between a voluntary home-like setting and a total institution grow different ways of life.

Obviously hospital and halfway house present to those who live in them very different social milieus. Not so obvious is how and what each social milieu communicates to those who live in it. We have few ways of asking about the effects of a given social atmosphere, and a questionnaire to halfway house directors—even if we had, as we do not, precise enough language to ask the right questions—is unlikely to produce the right result. Our dilemma here is that the major impact of the halfway house on its residents very likely comes from the milieu it provides, but the concept of milieu is so crude, so shapeless, so immense, and so uninvestigated that our explorations are blocked at the start—particularly from such simple, verbal methods as the questionnaire. What we have to say, then, derives mostly from clinical illustrations. The illustrations we use are, of course, selective. Our hope is that they nevertheless convey some of the flavor of what goes on.

As pointed out in Chapter 2 the term "therapeutic" milieu and its twin "therapeutic community," have been so abused that they are justifiably suspect. What is not suspect is the plain fact that environments do influence people. And if they do, possibly some environments are better than others for effecting a course of social adaptation to the ordinary requirements and opportunities of the community one lives in. The structure of the mental hospital milieu fosters adaptation to the world of the hospital. Critics have argued that such adaptation has little, and possibly negative, relevance for adaptation to the world outside the hospital. But with this latter world halfway houses are concerned. In their physical and household arrangements they recognize this world. Their emphases tend to be not so much on adaptation to life within the house but to life outside the house. We have seen this in their approaches to social activities, to work and to therapy.

And yet, were the halfway house only to emulate other community structures, it would offer little hope for improving the lives of those who have been severely damaged by the vicissitudes of life. The residents of halfway houses have suffered breakdown or have been on the edge of breakdown in the course of living in their communities. The halfway house is not simply a return to the community. It may be cousin to the boarding house or to the residential hotel, but these seldom offer psychological refuge to the disturbed.[2] The halfway house differs in presuming the function as a psychological resource; its acknowledged orientation is toward promoting the resident's transition to the community. Such an orientation presumes that the resident himself is not quite ready to enter fully into community life but that he can be helped in this process by living in the house.

In each of the preceding chapters we have been talking about the social milieus of halfway houses. Each description of a house represents, in a sense, a description of some aspects of its social environment and though we may question whether a term as inclusive as "milieu," can be at all useful, we can profitably look more closely at some of the components which go into making a social environment.

Fritz Redl (1959b) has attempted to do this. Although his analysis of components included in the concept of a therapeutic milieu is directed toward residential work with children, it is also appropriate here. Redl describes some twelve components. We comment on only a selected few of these, noting those aspects which relate to halfway houses.

The Social Structure of the Halfway House

A major facet of the social environment is, of course, the social structure. The social structure of the halfway house is determined, among other things, by: its size—rarely more than 30 and most often around 10 residents; its ecological setting and architecture—usually in the urban community and homelikes; its administrative structure and role distributions—usually that of simple rather than multiple subordination patterns. Such factors alone have direct impact on what goes on in the halfway house:

[2] Sociological studies have suggested that these institutions are more often the breeding grounds for pathology, though whether as cause or effect is by no means clear.

> At dinner one night after there had been some bickering between a pro- and an anti-TV faction, the pro-TV group decided to convert some basement space into its headquarters and leave the living room to the others. A staff member joined the enthusiastic TV viewers, took them in her car for paint and other decorating materials, and by 11:00 p.m. Woodley House had a newly decorated TV room in the basement and no further arguments with the others. No staff meeting or decisions were required; no requisition forms needed to be filled out; no cooling period elapsed between the idea and its execution (p. 284).

In the above quote from Rothwell and Doniger (1963) we may note: (1) the group is small enough to enable discussion and decision; (2) it is located in a house with living room and basement, etc., and with which the residents are sufficiently identified to be concerned with decoration; (3) the ecological setting is such that resources—in this case, paint and decorating materials—are easily available, but they must be sought outside the house and through contact with the community; (4) the problem is a practical one of comfort and convenience, not a matter of formal rules and regulations; (5) communication is direct and simple; (6) a staff member who had decision-making power is immediately involved; (7) the staff member is not limited by the prescribed definition of "professional" role; (8) action can be direct and immediate.

Because the structure of the halfway house is relatively simple, changes are relatively simple. A Harvard student who worked at Wellmet comments: "The students at Wellmet, because they are living in the house, spend a great deal of time there and, in fact, serve as the major agents of change. What do they change? They change the total milieu. How? By saying, 'Now we'll do it in a new way,' or 'let's forget about that rule' (Bennett, 1964, p. 21)."

How the structure of roles in a halfway house can be modified to suit the needs of a particular resident is illustrated by Kantor and Gelineau (Wellmet Progress Report, 1963):

> The resident had been hospitalized for ten years and out of the labor force for fifteen years. Because of his experiences prior to

and as a result of hospitalization, it was felt, on his admission, that the house social system would have to provide:

(a) counter-insulating experiences and opportunities;

(b) an expansion of the patient's role set, in order to expose him to higher role expectations;

(c) an elastic and flexible social control system calculated to facilitate his autonomy and independence;

(d) a human environment in which esteem-giving rather than degrading experiences were available; and

(e) a status system which offered the opportunity to rise in the system (p. 7).

After some initial unsuccessful efforts at conventional vocational counseling, planning was undertaken for a graduated program of pre-vocational training. The program was designed to ". . . utilize the processes available within the house social system to deal with the specific dynamic problems resulting from [the resident's] previous problems and hospitalization." All residents, both ex-patients and students, are ordinarily expected to assume some housekeeping duties. After some months the new resident was asked to *oversee* maintenance and repairs. Several months later when renovation of the house was undertaken, he was *placed in charge* of wallpapering and painting, a position which required him to supervise the work of others in the house and to deal with outside persons such as paint dealers and tool rental agencies. Sometime later a position was specifically created and assigned to the resident—that of budget manager:

This requires that [the resident] allocate funds for day-to-day expenses, make decisions as to the legitimacy of any expenses proposed by any other house members, deal directly with the administrators of the project, and accept responsibility for both the use of funds and the keeping of accurate records. This places him in a status and role approximating that of a productive and responsible male in any household, a role he has not been required to fulfill for the last fifteen years. These important maneuvers are aimed at helping him to overcome the subtle assaults that have been made upon his esteem and to restablish his masculine self-image. The stress we have put upon him is great. He is not expected to succeed immediately or without difficulty. Nevertheless, during the few months that [the resident] has been a member of the house, he has been able to overcome his long-standing dependence on the protectiveness of the custodial hospital and to support a greatly accelerated and extended range of interaction and responsibility. The plan now is to provide both support and additional social experiences in order to facilitate [the resident's] successful adaptation to the new and more demanding performance expected of him and to set the foundations for his resumption of a fulltime productive role in the work force and in the community.

The communication network of the halfway house, relatively simple compared with the complex one of the hospital, enables necessary changes to be made without great administrative lag. Furthermore, the manipulations and playing-off of staff members against one another that are so common in patient-staff relations in hospitals are more easily avoided or dealt with in the simpler communication structure of the halfway house.

The Value System of the Halfway House

Another component of the social milieu noted by Redl is the value system. Many of our earlier comments have suggested that the structural differences between halfway houses and hospitals derive from differences in values. And although halfway house directors do not all share the same values, there are certain emphases which they generally share. One of these is an antibureaucratic bias. Another is a positive concern for individuality and autonomy. We can understand why halfway house personnel have these values in common when we recall that halfway houses were often founded by people who rejected the hierarchical structure of mental hospitals and who sought more individualized patterns of work for themselves and of living for the mentally disturbed. The house structure allows staff to move beyond usual role definitions—to be themselves and to exercise their own tastes and talents. It allows them to treat residents and their problems individually—the range extending from dealing with pathology, through vocational planning (as seen in the example above), through the individualization of rules, to helping in everyday routines of living. Meal planning can, for example, take the individual tastes of residents into account; birthdays can be celebrated; shopping trips can be matched to the recreational or educational needs of particular residents.

Values are directed toward practical matters of the present rather than toward intrapsychic issues or the past. Not because halfway houses reject theoretical notions of individual psychodynamics or of psychotherapy; as we have seen psychotherapy is generally encouraged. But usually issues of traditional treatment are separated from the function of the halfway house. It is with the exigencies of everyday life that halfway houses concern themselves. Emphasis thus tends to be placed on action rather than fantasy and on adequate functioning rather than psychodynamic motivation:

> In many subtle and overt ways, residents are denied the "patient" identity. This is in contrast to hospitals where people are often pressed into accepting the idea of being a "patient." Some people are reluctant to give up the privileges and allowances made for them as patients. One man behaved in a particularly nasty fashion and then offered a long and brilliant psychiatric explanation for his behavior. He said in effect that he felt very badly and that his behavior was a function of his illness. I said, "Maybe you're sick, but you're nasty too, and it's not the same thing" (Doniger, 1964).

> . . . I said, "When you tell me you're hysterical about going to a job and typing, I'm not interested, but when you ask me to test you and see how fast you can type and I do, I have learned something and I'm interested. When you tell me you are preoccupied with thoughts of death, it interests me less than the thought that we are playing chess and you can beat me" (Rothwell & Doniger, 1966, p. 53).

One danger is of superficiality of approach. Halfway houses do not seem, however, to have succumbed to the temptations of a shallow pseudo-common sense. Probably the residents themselves are so disturbed that easy recourses and superficial theories meet with little success. But also those responsible for the direction of halfway houses often bring to their work considerable experience with the disturbed and considerable psychological sophistication; moreover, the common emphasis on consultation suggests there is a constant review of policies and actions.

The bias toward promoting adaptation to the community does, of course, suggest middle-class value systems, and in their operation halfway houses are likely to run according to middle-class standards. Their dependence on community support and their sensitivity to local neighborhood opinion fosters the middle-class orientation; it is probable, too, that most staff members come from middle-class backgrounds. Still, the emphasis on the immediate aspects of living fits in with nonmiddle-class values and is likely to be more comprehensible than the traditional psychotherapy model to those residents and their relatives who come from lower socioeconomic groups.

One other attitude which halfway houses seem to share is, as previous discussions have implied, a bias toward humanism. Joan Doniger puts it simply:

> Even on inevitable days when one tends to question his accomplishments I always was confident that, whatever its faults, life for most residents was better in Woodley House than in a hospital. Just because someone is diagnosed as schizophrenic, he should not have to eat institutional food the rest of his life, be regimented at meals and other times, or be shut out of kitchens and grocery stores. His enjoyment of good food and freedom may not treat or cure him— but it may make life better and that's what Woodley House is really about (1964).

The Rules and Rituals of Halfway Houses

Rules, rituals, routines, and standards are other parts of a social environment. As described in Chapter 10, the halfway house approach to them tends to be informal, ad hoc, and stylistically familial. They derive often from resident consensus rather than from staff imposition. A discussion of the handling of discipline is taken from the recent book by Rothwell and Doniger (1966):

> . . . What emerges from the [staff diary] descriptions is an impression of diversity—one person admonished as a child would be,

another counseled or advised as a college student might be, a third spoken to as a friend might be, a fourth encouraged, a fifth ignored.

Other impressions may also be obtained in the descriptions. People are dealt with directly, immediately and in terms of their present behavior . . . (p. 89).

The Staff is not consistently wise nor successful in its attempts at discipline. There are bickering, nagging, bad feelings and involvement where some objective and wise therapist in the same situation might be able to maintain equanimity and detachment. Staff moralizes and argues. Residents bait, complain and argue. On the other hand, there is little of the apathy, hopelessness and stagnancy often found in patient populations. People are engaged with each other and, if only tentatively or reluctantly, with life in the real world (p. 91).

The relative lack of standard routines is illustrated in another example from Woodley House:

The only continuing group activity for residents of Woodley House is eating dinner together. Everyone gets up at a different time and makes his own breakfast and almost everyone is away at midday. Other than the fixed dining hour, group activities wax and wane as residents come and go and change the atmosphere of the house. For example, when the temporary and part-time staff assistant changed —from a group worker to a history major—the atmosphere changed, too. About a year ago there was a very cohesive resident group and strong house spirit, with the residents sharing many activities—trips, picnics, swimming, concerts, movies, bowling. They formed a French class and brought a teacher into the house. Now residents do less together and many find friendships outside the house (Rothwell & Doniger, 1963, p. 282).

Other halfway houses may be somewhat more standardized in their programs and daily routines, but all contrast greatly with the hospital where schedules, rituals, and rules are fixed.

Space, Time, and "Props" in the Halfway House

An aspect of the social milieu greatly emphasized by Redl is the use of space, time, and objects. Unlike hospital space, halfway house space is open. Transition is between rooms rather than wards and offices, and movement is generally free, bounded only by common standards of family privacy. Transition between house boundaries and outside is also generally easy and convenient. Time, too, is "real" time. Waking and sleeping hours tend to be set by ordinary communal demands rather than by arbitrary rule. But a more interesting difference between halfway houses and hospitals is in their use of objects. The availability of equipment and objects of common use makes possible interactions inconceivable in the antiseptic hospital environment:

> A symmetrical relationship—you pin my hem, I pin yours; you cook the meat and I make the dessert; the house has a phonograph and I supply some new records—is possible when staff can see residents consistently as people and when residents have the opportunity to see staff at as close range as they are seen. Though it may be partly a function of ideology, the relationship between staff and residents . . . is possible in a halfway house because they live in the same real world. Residents have jobs as staff members do. They ride the same buses in the same traffic to and from work. They go to the same theatres and shop in the same stores. At home they cook in the same kitchen, eat in the same dining room and share the same bathrooms. Having so much in common, and so few situations which might perpetuate distance, ability to consider [the resident] a peer rather than a patient was fostered (Rothwell & Doniger, 1966, p. 61).

These "props" of ordinary life can function in two ways. First, residents who have been dissociated from the community can begin to learn or relearn to handle the ordinary complexities of the typical world of objects in the community. Staff can assist them in this learning in a simple and natural way. Residents can be helped in the common tasks of handling money, kitchen and laundry equipment, transportation facilities. Most often such assistance is casual, given as problems and questions arise:

> I woke [the resident] up late in the morning and we went grocery shopping. She's excited about life outside the hospital; about grocery stores, about how to cook beets, and about all the ordinary details, but she's inept about work and has to be taught things that most

people can figure out, like how to open cans or turn pancakes. Grocery shopping and putting the cans into the shopping basket delighted her. At supper she announced that my day would have been a lot harder if she hadn't been there to help me push the cart and do the dishes (Rothwell & Doniger, 1966, p. 36).

Assistance can also be planned and intensive as, for example, in Fountain House's program of helping residents adjust to new jobs.

The second way in which common objects serve is as settings for interactions around a personal issue:

> While doing the dishes [the resident] started to talk about the man she dates. She said that neither of them is serious and she doesn't want to get serious until she's well. She also talked about someone else she likes who was a fellow patient. He seems to be a lot sicker than she. Then she started to talk about her family. She went upstairs and brought down pictures of her sisters and parents and described all of them. I got the impression from her conversation that she is her mother's favorite and when I suggested that, she was surprised and pleased: "How did you know?" She said that her father was very strict . . . (Rothwell & Doniger, 1966, p. 30).

> We were in the kitchen and, although this was the first time she'd talked with me at Woodley House, she remembered I'd been at the hospital where she was a patient, and talked freely, as if I knew her well. She was telling me about her mother's many talents—particularly how well she sewed and how she'd made all of her daughters' dresses. This reminded her that she needed to take up the hem on a dress for tomorrow. So I pinned the hem and she spent the rest of the evening sewing (Rothwell & Doniger, 1966, p. 31).

Those who work with young children are well aware that children can often sustain a serious or intimate conversation far better when clinician and child are occupied in a task involving an object which can serve as a focus of distraction from the intensity of an issue. Toys, tools, mild craft or athletic activities, so long as they are not fully preoccupying, can serve such a purpose. For adults also an interpersonal situation without props can be too threatening—either because of the topic or the relation—to be productive. To tolerate the object bareness of the usual adult psychotherapy situation demands both strong motivation and firm ego capacities. Even mature adults have their props—cigarette, pipe, paper and pencil, knitting, whittling—to tide them over difficult moments. A shared task like washing dishes, sewing, ironing, garden work, painting, or carpentry can enable interpersonal discussions in the halfway house which would not otherwise occur.

Interactions and the "Life Space Interview" in Halfway Houses

We are thus led into the most important part of the social environment—what goes on between people. We have little specific information to offer here on what goes on among house residents. Certainly interactions and changes in resident interaction in the course of a resident's career need to be studied. Though interactions between staff and resident have not been fully or systematically reported the illustrations above have been selected in part because they suggest some potentialities for staff-resident interchange. Here we would again refer to a paper by Redl (1959a). Commenting on relations between adults and children, he conceptualizes and describes some strategies and techniques of the *life space interview.* Though they have not yet been subject to formalization or technical discussion, such interviews play an important part in the lives of all children. They occur whenever an issue of a child's direct life experience becomes a focus for discussion between child and adult. The issue may be an immediate one—helping a child deal with a hurt, or handle a fight with another child, or tolerate a delay in momentary gratification, or deal with the emotional impact of anger, anxiety, panic, guilt or shame. Or it may be a more long-standing issue of concern. Such interviews, whether or not one thinks of them as such, and whether or not they are helpful or destructive, occur constantly between parents and children and between teachers and children. They present special opportunities not only for encouragement and support, for necessary—in Redl's terms—"emotional first aid on the spot," but also for what he calls the "clinical exploitation of life events."

Much of what occurs between staff and residents in half-way houses fits the concept of *life space interview*. Though there are probably fewer issues requiring emotional first aid for halfway house residents than there are for children in average households, they are by no means lacking:

> A very upset young girl was weeping one morning. When asked what was bothering her, she said her therapist had forbidden her to go to church. A staff member immediately phoned the girl's therapist, then asked her to speak on the extension in a three-way conversation. It soon became apparent that the doctor had mildly suggested that if going to church upset the girl, she might try staying home one Sunday. With this clarification of the real dilemma, the staff member was able to help the resident make up her mind about going to church (Rothwell & Doniger, 1963, p. 284).

There are many opportunities to utilize life events toward a goal of clinical change. One of the above illustrations, in which a resident attempted to exploit a psychiatric explanation for his behavior and evoked from the staff person in reply, "Maybe you're sick, but you're nasty too, and it's not the same thing," represents one such possibility. The staff member's response is in no way naive. Rather it illustrates an attempt at what Redl calls *symptom estrangement*. The staff person is aware that the resident's explanation is a defensive maneuver designed to protect him from responsibility for the consequences of his actions. She responds to him in such a way as to point out that the explanation itself is a "symptomatic" distortion, thus helping him become aware of how he misuses his "illness."

More often events between resident and staff person provide an opportunity to point up reality issues and to help the resident differentiate what is real from what is fantasy:

> [A resident is upset because a stranger had tried to pick her up during her lunch hour. She talks about this with one of the halfway house staff. The staff member notes]: She told him she didn't want to be picked up. She talked this incident over with her social worker but

still felt upset. I said, to console her, that some things which happen are not reflections of ourselves. If someone tried to pick you up, it doesn't mean that it's your fault or that you are to blame. The resident said this was very helpful and comforting and she felt much better . . . (Rothwell & Doniger, 1966, pp. 30–31).

As she was leaving, she said, "If I ever got to be a social worker or doctor or something like that, I would always encourage people to be what they want to be." I answered, "Well, you'll never get indiscriminate encouragement from me." She said that my comment had changed her whole life. I said I didn't see why. Modest and possible goals make the most sense to me but if I were wrong, she could prove that she could be a psychiatrist. Again, she repeated that she had the talent and intelligence to be a psychiatrist. I agreed that she might, but it seemed a hard task to set for herself . . . (Rothwell & Doniger, 1966, p. 50).

Then she said, "You know, I have another solution. When I have the urge to go to the bridge, you come with me." She said this with her eyes shining as if it were a wonderful idea. I replied, "That's the most ghoulish idea you've ever had." She was very surprised by my reaction. People usually go along with her theatrical notions but I said, "Any time you want to jump off the bridge, go by yourself. I won't be party to that kind of wild and sick action." Then I repeated that her life was not worth anything in anybody else's hands (Rothwell & Doniger, 1966, pp. 52–53).

An illustration from Rutland Corner House:

. . . One woman was very pleased when Miss Grant [the Director] showed no alarm at her taking 20 aspirins: "She said she would do what she could to help me and she thought milk would be good to drink" (Landy & Greenblatt, 1965, p. 26).

Life in the halfway house presents daily opportunities, under natural circumstances, for staff to make counter-illusory efforts. Staff also have opportunities to offer residents new ways of dealing with events and new ways of looking at themselves:

A resident goes for a job interview. The staff member reports: When she returned after the interview, she told me all the things about it that were wrong, but neglected to say that she was offered the job. I pointed out that, whether or not she wanted the job, it was flattering that he wanted her (Rothwell & Doniger, 1966, p. 40).

Far too little reasearch has been done on the interventions which are part of everyday life. A study by Goodrich and Boomer (1958) examined critical incidents occurring between staff and children in residential treatment. The study yielded 31 classes of staff transactions which were further grouped under four super-ordinate headings: (*a*) promoting personality change by helping the child to view his own behavior evaluatively; (*b*) promoting ego growth; (*c*) supporting existing ego controls; and (*d*) managing one's own conduct as a staff person. Redl and Wineman (1951, 1952) and Redl in his other writings (1966) also give vivid illustrations of staff-child interactions, and they also present functional classifications of the events between staff and children. Nothing comparable exists for what goes on in halfway houses, although the illustrations presented by Rothwell and Doniger (1966) are a significant beginning.

The Resiliency Potential of the Halfway House

By virtue of its simple structure, the halfway house can respond resiliently to its residents' problems and needs. This potentiality for rapid response according to circumstances is another facet of the social environment of the halfway house which makes it different from the hospital:

> They [the residents] feel she [the Director] has understanding and appreciate her skill in "handling situations" . . . they don't feel that she intrudes on their privacy but are confident that she is at hand if needed . . . (Landy & Greenblatt, 1965, p. 26).

Intimate studies of halfway house social environments are few. Certainly far more studies are needed to capture the atmosphere of what goes on in the great variety of conditions which half-way houses represent. The "critical incidents" we have cited convey a flavor. The flavor is very different from that of even the best hospital. It is different from that of a typical boarding house. It suggests the uniqueness of the halfway house as an institution.

Chapter 14   LEAVING THE
            HALFWAY HOUSE

THE GOAL SET BY MOST HALFWAY HOUSES FOR THE RESIDENT IS THE
traditional one of independent functioning and self-support in the
community. The structure of the house, the expectations of the
staff, and presumably the hopes and plans of the resident are all
geared to this prospect. The last several chapters convey something
of the intensity of efforts expended toward this goal. Presumably,
then, success for the halfway house is tokened by its residents' assumption of normal life in the broader social community. In practice the matter is somewhat more complicated.

Time of Stay

The average resident does not remain very long at the halfway house (Table 10). Although six houses describe the average
period of residence as a year or more, the median length of stay falls
between four and eight months for the 34 houses reporting.[1]
Data on average length of residence yield little knowledge
about the considerations and problems of termination. Who is to
decide just when the proper time and conditions have been achieved

[1]Six halfway houses claimed that they were too recently established to
provide data.

TABLE 10. Stated Average Length of
Resident Stay

	Number of Houses
4 months and under	11
4 to 8 months	11
8 to 12 months	6
One year or more	6
House too new	6
	40

—the individual himself, the therapists, the house staff, or an intricate balance of all these at some point coming to a consensus? A questionnaire item inquiring about the responsibility for this decision unfortunately yielded little differentiable information. It is apparent, however, that houses differ considerably on the issues affecting termination decisions.

Some, particularly if there is a close connection with a hospital and there are people waiting to come to the halfway house, set an arbitrary time limit which is made known to incoming residents. If there are limits, they are usually set within a year, at three, six, nine, or twelve months. Houses which fix a time limit believe that such definition acts to encourage the resident's orientation toward independence and to enhance his progress in the time allotted to him. Staffs of other houses believe there may be destructive effects from inflexible cut-off dates; they prefer to wait for the time when the resident feels ready to leave. Many houses are in a category between these two; they make no specific stipulation as to when a resident should leave, but if after a certain length of time he is still hazy about future plans, concern becomes more pointed. Staff initiates discussion about departure and even sets a particular time limit on his further residence.

All houses concerned with fostering transition to community have some way of encouraging departure. Encouragements range from setting firm departure dates, as noted above, to subtle suggestions. One house uses its fee schedule—increasing fees quite noticeably after one year—to provide an added push. The experience of another house is that residents who have not begun to take steps toward planning by their second month at the house are not likely to do so by themselves and require more active staff help. Still another house schedules a meeting in the third month of each resident's stay to talk about his future. Where planning has been nonexistent or sketchy and help is required, the staff finds a way to provide it. Such help may be primarily practical—apartment finding, help with moving, etc.—or it may be a continued emphasis on support and encouragement. Whatever the specific technique, there is always the atmosphere of expectation, the implicit presumption that each person *will* move out.

Residents do not necessarily have to be encouraged or pressured to leave the halfway house. In relation to Rutland Corner House, where it is mostly the resident herself who initiates the move—usually at about six months—Landy and Greenblatt (1965) note a number of intrinsic reasons which influence the urge toward departure:

(1) They feel they will be asked to leave soon in any event, and "might as well get out while there are still good feelings all around."

(2) Their friends usually have already left. Several former residents live near Rutland Corner House. They drop in frequently to visit their friends and/or Miss Grant. And there is much visiting by residents with friends who have already established themselves on the outside. Two of the women were so close to friends on the outside who had nearby apartments that they spent more time in their friends' residences than in the House.

(3) They find the newer, sicker women increasingly difficult to live with. Thus when Nancy was coming in, Gloria, who had known Nancy on the ward, said, "If they send her here, I'm leaving to get a place of my own." Another remarked about a rather disturbed sister-resident, "I've got a job, I don't have to stay around and watch her stare into space." These attitudes further help to explain initial reactions to new residents noted earlier.

(4) The older resident will begin to show signs of wanting to drop the "sick" role, and its most recent association, namely, the halfway

house. Said one, "I shall always feel like a patient as long as I'm living with other patients—which you have to do at Rutland Corner House."

(5) As the resident begins to make friends on the job, or elsewhere on the outside, she grows uneasy that they may discover where she lives. Or she may want a place of her own, where she can relax, "be myself" and "entertain friends" (pp. 90–91).

Where Residents Go On Leaving

Each of the 40 facilities was asked where residents went on leaving the house and the approximate percentage for the various alternatives (Table 11). Since ten houses felt they had had insufficient experience to give a meaningful reply, and since five more failed to answer the item or give percentage values which did not add up accurately, only 25 usable replies were obtained. In considering these responses, it became apparent that the VA-affiliated houses (N=7) and the non-VA-connected houses (N=18) presented different patterns of movement into the community. The difference in these patterns is visible in Table 11.

TABLE 11. Where Residents Go On Leaving the House

	VA Houses (N=7) %	Non-VA Houses (N=18) %
Return to the hospital within the year	18.00	19.00
Return to their families	37.00	11.30
Go to a foster home situation	17.00	4.00
Live independently in the community	27.00	59.90
Other	1.00	1.30
Not ascertained	.00	4.50
	100.00	100.00

Houses associated with the VA tend to return residents to their own families to a greater extent—a reported average of 37%—than do non-VA-houses—an average of 11%. Residents of VA-affiliated houses seem more likely (17%) than residents of non-VA houses (4%) to be placed in a foster home facility. It should be recognized here that foster home placement is very often reserved for those who, it is felt, cannot make a fuller adjustment to community living. The people so placed are often those considered as having low rehabilitation and employment potential, but not so badly off as to require continuous hospital care. Almost 20% of the residents of both VA and non-VA facilities must return to hospitals. The major difference between VA and non-VA houses is in the average percentages of residents whom they report as leaving to live independently in the community, which non-VA houses claim as 60%, VA houses only 27%. Overall, residents who leave the halfway house tend predominantly to move into living independently in the community.

The percentages cannot, of course, tell a full story. As is true of discharge rates, the disposition of those residents who leave is likely to be at least in part a function of the initial selection process. Those houses taking more disturbed or more chronic ex-patients are likely to show different patterns of resident disposition from those who take ex-patients of only high rehabilitative potential. For such percentages to be fully meaningful, adequately controlled studies would be required.

Post-Departure Relationships

The follow-up of the ex-resident may be considered in terms of two sets of functions. Follow-up may be thought of as part of the clinical process, whereby the resident's relation with the house is eased off rather than broken off, and whereby the process of adjustment to the community can be facilitated even though the resident has left the house. The second function is that of a research appraisal of how well the house is accomplishing its aims.

The actual break from the house need not be sharp. The move itself, as Landy and Greenblatt (1965) suggest, may be stretched over several days, and the former resident who lives close by may visit often in the first few months. It is clear from the questionnaire replies that most houses place emphasis on a continuing relationship with the resident for some period after he has left the house. For example, only two of the 36 houses replying to an item on visits said they did not encourage visits from ex-residents. The promotion of visits is apparently successful since at least some ex-residents tended to visit in all houses where this was encouraged. Furthermore, although respondents were not queried on the subject, it is apparent (Woodley House Conference, 1963) that a number of houses have worked out intermediate arrangements with some of their ex-residents. One of these is to allow or encourage the resident to continue boarding at the halfway house after he has left it. Fountain House encourages the ex-residents of its apartments to continue in its extensive and diversified program of social and recreational activities.

Similarly, in response to another questionnaire item, 31 ' ɔuses said that there was some form of follow-up of ex-residents, and only 5 said there was none. Those claiming follow-up mostly seemed to be referring to it as parts of the clinical process. For example, VA houses generally referred the ex-resident to a conveniently located VA clinic. The most general form of follow-up was by nonsystematic social or semi-social contacts. These could vary from invitations to visit on special occasions to such things as letters, telephone calls, and Christmas cards. It is likely that such procedures are highly selective, and that there is considerable selectivity in the residents who respond to them. Data on follow-up presented in Table 12 reveal only eight houses had a formal and somewhat systematic procedure for follow-up. These involved definite procedures for contacting all residents, though how persistent the efforts and how adequate the procedures are not known. Several houses currently have research programs which include follow-up. As far as is known, only two of these, Fountain House and Conard House, employ control groups, matched to the resident population, for follow-up study. A survey of eight California half-way houses suggests that residents want some continued contact after leaving and suggests ways of meeting these needs (Shaw, 1965).

TABLE 12. Follow-Up

	Number of Houses
Follow-Up	
A formal procedure	8
Non-systematic or social follow-up	14
Through on-going therapy	3
Through VA clinics or offices	6
No Follow-Up	
Previously did study	1
Planning study	1
Reason not given	3
Too early—not enough residents have left	4
	40

Problems of Separation: The Premature Leaver and the Permanent Resident

We noted that the average length of halfway house residence was between four and eight months. There are, of course, residents who leave after a shorter period. Some of these are from houses with a three-month limit. Others are capable of rapid adjustment to the requirements of life in the outside community. But some of the early departures represent "failures" of the house. In this latter group are those, perhaps mis-selected for the particular house, who must—often within the month after admission to the house—return to the hospital. The group includes also those who, for one reason or another, decide to quit the house. They may reject the values, the social atmosphere, or the work emphasis of the house. Such residents may return to family or find independent housing. They often lack employment and must depend on family, pension, or welfare support. Thus, not all who leave within a short time represent positive effects of experience in halfway houses. Gumrukcu and Mikels (1965) suggest that for Conrad House those staying less than two months are likely to represent failures of the House in its selection or function.

At the other end of the scale are those residents who remain in the house indefinitely. The problem does not arise where houses have and enforce a fixed time limit; residents either find other accommodations or return to the hospital. But where there is no firmly kept time boundary and where funds are available to maintain the resident in the house, it is possible for him to become a permanent member. Responses to the questionnaire item which asked whether any residents stayed indefinitely at the house indicate that for 17 of the 38 houses replying the issue of the permanent resident is salient. The problem for staff then becomes what to do about it, and how best even to think about it.

One side of the problem is its effect on the staff and the house. The issue here is a general one. It arises for any person or agency providing a clientele with services of long or indefinite duration. Under such circumstances the development of a "hardcore" group is inevitable. That is, purely on the basis of mathematical probabilities, length of connection between agency and clinetele will progress toward its maximum time limit. In the halfway house, for example, if "successful" cases leave and "unsuccessful" ones stay, and some proportion of newly admitted residents are likely to be "unsuccessful", the houses where there are no time pressures will become increasingly filled with permanently "unsuccessful" cases. Staff morale is likely to be lowered by the continuing presence of these residents because they represent to the staff their "failures." Also, long-term living with the same residents may prove irksome and unchallenging, particularly to those who are motivated by therapeutic aims, as are most halfway house personnel. Furthermore, permanent residence may prove contagious. Movement from the house is difficult even for those most ready, and the temptations offered by the example of the permanent resident may reduce incentives for taking this step. Those houses which acknowledge this problem handle it variously; in general there seems to be little consensus or feeling of satisfaction with attempted solutions. One house has, as noted, used a boost in fees after a year's residence to encourage departure. Other houses have different built-in devices, apart from time limits, for keeping residents moving. For example, at the Vermont Rehabilitation Houses there were initially long waiting lists. All residents were aware of this and consequently felt pressured to leave in order to give others a turn.[2]

We have been looking at that side of the problem which has to do with staff and house needs. But there is another side. This has to do with resident and community needs. The issues are general ones for rehabilitative services. They are stated cogently by Beard and Goldman (1964):

> First of all, is there a need for a community facility especially designed for the long-term patient whose adjustment in the community may be dependent upon his continued participation in the setting? Are these not patients who would have to return to the hospital were it not for such settings? Should we be comfortable in having such patients return to the hospital rather than provide special community programs for them? Should we not pursue our efforts to find in the community the kind of sustaining influences that the patient requires rather than have him return to the hospital to find such supports?

> The same problem can be approached from another point of view. How certain are we that the patient's continuation in our program is primarily indicative of his own inability to achieve a higher level of functioning? Might it be, rather, indicative of our own inability to provide him with the special kind of rehabilitative procedures which will help maintain and develop his community adjustment?

[2] But even here the situation has changed with time. To the extent that these houses have been successful in rehabilitating hospital patients, waiting lists have shortened and the residents no longer feel so much pressure. Furthermore, since the most promising candidates were selected early, the residents entering at a later point tend to have a somewhat lower potential for complete rehabilitation; thus a "hard-core" population has been developing and movement of the residents out of the houses has been more difficult to achieve than it used to be.

One additional point: We recognize that the community at present is unable to accommodate the "chronic" patient. Does this imply that it should not do so? We recognize that our society is clearly deficient in meeting the needs of various populations. Our solution hopefully is not that of constructing institutions apart from the local community, such as mental hospitals. If centers such as ours do not concern themselves with this special problem, what facility should (p. 15)?

What can be done to serve those residents who may never be able to live independently, but who do not require hospital security, remains a pressing problem for the halfway house administrator. Many houses *do* occasionally permit such residents to stay on a rather indefinite and relatively permanent basis.

The dilemma is not insoluble. And, in fact, halfway houses have begun to develop some innovative approaches to this matter of transition from halfway house to community. Some houses— notably Fountain House and Spring Lake Ranch—rather than thinking of movement solely in terms of individuals, have adopted the plan of moving out groups of residents who have functioned well together in the halfway house. At other houses such arrangements occur informally—two or more residents find and share an apartment. Through such groupings, residents can avoid the shock of finding themselves completely alone. They may be able to augment each other's abilities and thus may help to sustain one another through difficult periods in much the way a satisfactory family unit does. The permanence or transitoriness of such arrangements its a fertile area for exploration. It might be well to consider programs of group movement as part of a consciously planned design.[3]

A more common way of easing departure from the house is by making the break a gradual one, in either of two ways. The house can for a time encourage visits and participation in house social events by the newly separated former member. Or it can ease the transition by having the former resident live nearby but

---

[3] Fairweather (1964) suggests a similar possibility of movement in small groups for those leaving the mental hospital.

continue to board at the house. Many houses adopt one or both of these procedures. Either way the resident can retain the society and support of the house.

Landy and Greenblatt (1965) note that some 80% of former residents of Rutland Corner House continued to maintain some relation through visits, with 20% visiting two or more times a month. They go on to comment:

> The question may arise in the reader's mind as to whether this revisiting represents a type of "dependency" on the House. In the narrow sense of the word perhaps it does, but it does not seem to us that this is disproportionately more than any individual's attachment to the place and people with whom he has had meaningful experiences. One might speak of this as "mature" dependency, in the sense that often the forces that pull the former residents back to Rutland Corner House seem to spring not from pathological "one-way" dependency, but from normal desires to maintain old friendships, share new experiences, and receive the support and counsel of Miss Grant.

> Thus the transitional function of the House does not terminate with discharge, but tapers off gradually until the women have reached the stage, once in the community, when all their relationships are with "outsiders." Revisiting in this perspective represents an advanced stage in the process of personal growth and community restoration. It is as expectable for the former resident to continue to visit the House as for the former soldier to consort with his "buddies" in a veterans' organization, or for the former student to join his alumni association (p. 93).

One possible innovation, which, so far as we know, has not been used, would make it possible for residents to move from one halfway house to another instead of confining movement either to the community or to the mental hospital. The diversity in population, structural arrangements, and procedures among halfway houses makes it likely that residents misplaced in one house would fit better in another. Such a move might be undertaken to benefit either the resident or the staff, or simply because of a time deadline. Some residents who are becoming permanent in one environment may respond better in another; staff may also require a change. One participant at the Woodley House Conference offered as a solution to the progressive "hard-core" problem the not altogether facetious suggestion that at a certain point in halfway house existence staff rather than residents might move out, leaving the residents together as a coherent functioning group.

One possibility is to give up the goal of complete independence for those unable to achieve it. Permanent, semicustodial "quarter-way" houses might be established. These houses would be similar to halfway houses in their functioning except that no one would be pressured to leave. Staff would not see the permanent resident as a personal failure. Here the more modest satisfactions of the improvement of life in the house over that in hospitals, the notion that "every day outside the hospital is a good day" would be stressed. Efforts would be devoted to avoiding the deterioration which takes place during long-term residence in a hospital. This accentuation of the positive element in the resident's having progressed as far as a half- or quarter-way house might have the virtue for both the staff and the resident of reducing the level of demand on those who cannot tolerate the strain of high expectations and possible failure. A few of the rural houses take a view similar to this, expressing little or no concern about the length of time spent in the "good life" they offer. There is no inherent logical reason for insisting that the house perform a transitional function for *all* residents. For some, the halfway, quarter-way or three-quarter-way house might offer a permanent solution considerably more satisfactory than a continued hospital existence.

Part

IV

THE FUTURE
OF
HALFWAY
HOUSES

Chapter 15   SUMMARY, IMPLICATIONS,
             AND PROSPECTS

Summary

IN THE FIVE YEARS AFTER THE 1958 SURVEY OF HALFWAY HOUSES
for the mentally disturbed (Wechsler, 1960), the number of halfway houses increased five-fold. There appears to be no abatement
but rather an intensification of this trend. Such rapid growth reflects
a need and an attempt to develop resources to meet this need. Preceding chapters of this book discuss the forces converging to create
this need and the influences which led to the development of halfway houses.

The halfway house is one of a number of newly developing
transitional facilities. It is a residential institution designed with
the ostensible goal of effecting the transition of the ex-patient from
the mental hospital to the community. The idea is simple enough.
Yet a more precise definition is necessary. For, if we are to consider
the potentialities and limitations of the halfway house movement,
we need details. We need to know how halfway houses are structured and how they work.

For this purpose, a questionnaire was developed and sent
to all facilities which might possibly meet some generally accepted
criteria which define halfway houses for the mentally disturbed:
(*a*) that the residents have recognized psychiatric problems; (*b*)
that the halfway house is usually not on hospital grounds; (*c*) that

it is, if only temporarily, the primary residence of the persons living there; (*d*) that presumably the residents do not remain permanently. The forty institutions which replied to the questionnaire are close to a total sample of the situation existing at the time of the study in mid-1963. The main body of this book derives from analysis of the replies, supplemented by information from published reports, brochures, conference materials, and personal exchange.

What emerges are, as might be expected, some commonalities and some diversities. A general portrait can be drawn of the halfway house career of that fiction, the modal resident of the modal halfway house:

> The modal resident of the modal halfway house is an exhospital patient, at one time diagnosed as schizophrenic. Directly or shortly after leaving the hospital, he came to the house, perhaps after some visiting. He finds the house very different from the hospital ward. For one thing it is in a residential area of the city. It is a many-roomed place, dating from the twenties or thirties, in town rather than in the suburbs. It is a house, and it looks like a house and not like a hospital. Aside from staff, there are only about ten other residents. The resident has his own room or he shares a room with just one other person; also, unlike the hospital, the house has no locked rooms. While there are lots of things to do at the house, he has to go outside for any special entertainment. Moreover, he pays for his room and board. These cost him about $90 a month [in 1963], a fee that covers little more than half of the expenses that the house requires for his care.

> At the modal house the resident receives no written rules. Still, he finds out that there are some things he must not do—such as drink on the premises, and some things that he must do—such as tell staff when he goes out, come to meals promptly, keep himself and the premises clean and obey his doctor's orders. He must care for his own room and he is usually expected to do some extra work of his own choice around the house. If he doesn't live up to these requirements, considerable social pressure will be placed on him and he may even be threatened with having to leave the house. In some ways then it isn't like living independently at a boarding house; it is much more closely supervised, and there is much more interaction

with staff and with other residents. But it isn't like a hospital either; for example, he doesn't have to get "passes," and no one threatens to remove his "privileges."

There are other ways in which the house is unlike a boarding house. For example, although the day-to-day management is by a non-professional staff, there is close professional direction and consultation by a non-resident staff, who are likely to be social workers, and there is also a board which guides policy. These arrangements operate to encourage the resident along various lines. For instance, chances are that he doesn't have a job. But some residents at the house have outside jobs which pay, and the house will expend efforts to motivate him and help him find work. If he gets a job, he manages his own income; if he is not yet ready or is unable to hold a paying job, the house will encourage him to undertake whatever volunteer work he is able to do. Another line along which he is encouraged, although it is not an absolute condition for continued residence, is therapy. His therapist, usually a psychiatrist, does not live at the house, but does consult informally with house staff.

The modal resident will stay at the house from four to eight months. When he leaves, it will probably be to live independently in the community [If, however, his house is sponsored by the Veterans Administration, he is more likely to return to his family.] After he leaves, the house will encourage him to visit. They may invite him to board at the house while living elsewhere if he wishes; in any case they will try to maintain some informal and unsystematic contact with him. He is, however, unlikely to be a subject in a research follow-up study.

The modal sketch suggests the characteristics which comprise a halfway house. Each of these characteristics is typical of one or another societal institution, but the particular combination is typical of none but the halfway house.

The halfway house is not a hospital. It differs from the hospital not only in many structural features, but also in the democratic, informal, and relaxed atmosphere it provides. In virtually every aspect of living, the resident assumes a far greater degree of autonomy than does the patient in a hospital. He is not forced into the fixed patterns required by a complex administrative hierarchy but can make decisions for himself. Yet in some respects the halfway house is like a hospital. It retains the rehabilitative aims of the hospital and the emphasis on therapeutic function.

The physical arrangements, for the most part, resemble those of a boarding house. Yet the halfway house is not quite a boarding house. One obvious difference is that the residents of the halfway house have similar problems and have undergone a similar history of hospitalization. Furthermore, in contrast with the boarding house landlady, the professionally directed halfway house staff is committed to an interest in the resident and to encouragement and support of his social and vocational adaptation to the community. In this commitment and through the influence of this commitment on the daily life of the resident, the halfway house differs from a boarding house or residential hotel. Certainly, too, the social anonymity possible in these latter institutions is impossible for the halfway house resident.

The halfway house situation is somewhat like family life in its informal atmosphere and style of living, in its demand for participation, and in the promise of comfort and support in difficult times. Yet it is unlike a family in being free from associations with past happenings in the resident's life: emotional involvements are less intense and in many cases less pathological. In the kinds of demands it makes and in the way it makes them the halfway house is different from the family. Commenting on Rutland Corner House, Landy and Greenblatt (1965) note:

> Miss Grant [the Director] does not see her role as a motherly one: ". . . The girls have had enough of mothers; they have problems to work out relating to their own mothers without my complicating the picture . . . I don't see that as my purpose" . . . The women do not usually speak of Miss Grant as a mother . . . They say she is "the best friend I ever had," . . . "like a sister, an older sister." (p. 26).

In some ways the halfway house resembles a small boarding school. They have in common the double function of education and protection. They are both, in a sense, transitional facilities, maintaining their function only until their charges achieve enough wisdom and independence to graduate.

Although the halfway house shares its features with those of other social institutions, only in the halfway house are these features found together. It is the combination which constitutes the uniqueness of the halfway house and its raison d'être, and in this combination the halfway house exemplifies the transitional function for which it was designed.

Helping to make the halfway house unique among institutions is its reflection of attitudes which regard its function as more than merely transitional. Not all halfway house personnel subscribe to all of these attitudes, but the following expressions are sufficiently shared to constitute a broad description:

1. A halfway house is a place for ex-hospitalized and/or upset people to live in order to avoid the necessity for hospitalization.

2. It is a place to live uncontaminated by the stigma of a hospital.

3. It is a place where the individual has more opportunity to influence his environment than in a larger more highly structured organization.

4. It is a place, free from association with past difficulties, and old intense relationships, which provides opportunities to readjust to societal norms over a period of time after hospitalization.

5. It provides the support which is necessary before people can find supports in other places.

6. It provides an arena for trying out different roles and behaviors.

7. It provides normal models for emulation and peers for comfort.

8. It encourages and even forces normal patterns of living and associations with the broader community.

9. It is a social system which is intentionally manipulated for the benefit of the resident population.

10. It is a place where mentally disturbed people can live with dignity and where they are provided with an atmosphere that is receptive to improvement.

These views—from the Woodley House Conference in 1963—are perhaps clues to a broader orientation which seems to characterize halfway house organizers. That orientation combines a strong anti-bureaucratic, individualistically-oriented bias with a rather middle-class ethos and with a practical down-to-earth outlook. And pervading this orientation is a deep humanistic commitment.

The modal house, based on "average" figures, is an abstraction and probably does not exist anywhere. What is more interesting and important is the picture of diversity presented by respondents. Wide ranges of difference were found in every aspect of the study. For example, the residence may be an apartment in a central metropolitan area or a farm far out in the country. It may be inhabited solely by men, solely by women, or by both men and women. Living in the house are ex-patients, but possibly also youth hostelers, normal college undergraduates, or transient guests. The house staff may refer to its population as patients, members, clients, or guests. A resident may never have been hospitalized, or he may have spent ten years or more on the back ward of a state hospital. During his stay at the house he may pay nothing or $700 a month. The staff in charge may belong to any of a number of different professions or to none at all. The resident may leave the house after a few weeks or he may stay permanently without any pressure to leave. These diversities suggest some general issues and highlight some potentialities.

Emerging from the diversity are images of two different models, representing countervailing tendencies which the structures of the houses reflect. The more traditional model, which might be called a "medical" model, is based on a rationale of illness and recuperation. In this model, the corrective process, "therapy," takes place outside the house. The house itself is seen primarily as a supporting or even neutral environment in which restorative processes are given time and opportunity to occur. But "cure" itself is not a function of the house.

A newer viewpoint, which might be called a "sociological" model, looks toward recent developments in social approaches to problems of mental disturbance, with an emphasis on social adaptation. In houses with this orientation, the house program *itself* is designed to play the major active role in corrective and restorative processes to help bring a resident to a satisfactory and productive life. Efforts are made to structure the house and modify processes of on-going events and relationships so as to produce conditions and provide experiences which, in themselves, effect significant changes in people. The principles guiding these programs are presumably derived from the body of knowledge and opinion in anthropology, psychiatry, psychology, social work, and sociology.

These concepts are exemplified in some recent innovations in mental hospitals and are receiving increasing consideration by those concerned with general problems of mental health. And since the administrative structure of the halfway house is considerably simpler than that of the mental hospital, and its processes are considerably less formal, a halfway house presents conditions for utilizing this approach flexibly. The model suggests, for example, that the house may change to fit the needs of the resident, rather than requiring the resident to change in order to fit the house. An illustration, more fully discussed in Chapter 13, describes this possibility:

> Mr. B., a passive dependent, middle-aged man who had suffered basic injury to his self-esteem and masculine self-image in early life, was, after a time, given two responsible positions in the House management. The first was the full responsibility for supervising and arranging a major redecoration project in the House. The second was as budget manager, a higher status position because it carried responsibility for allocating and keeping records of all day-to-day House funds . . . The demands of these positions on Mr. B. were great, but the conscious House plan was that everything possible would be done ". . . to facilitate Mr. B.'s successful adaptation to the new and more demanding performance expected of him and to set the foundation for his resumption of a full-time productive role in the work force and in the community" (Wellmet Progress Report, 1963).

In this example, there was recognition that greater efficiency would have been achieved by having a staff member undertake this responsibility. The aim, however, was to provide the resident with the opportunity to test himself in a responsible role and to allow him to learn and find satisfaction in this process. Such an experiment was judged more useful in the long run than would be the smooth operation of the House. Other observers have noted similarly that occasional crises may serve a useful function, sometimes helping residents to recognize their own unexplored capacities for constructive action in relation to their own lives and in relation to others. Once discovered, these potential strengths can be fostered.

The contrasting approaches represented by the medical and sociological models need not be wholly antithetical to one another. For example, within the sociological model, psychotherapy may be seen as necessary in order to enable capacities of the resident to emerge; the changes resulting from psychotherapy may empower the resident to use the influences which the house can provide. Alternatively, within the medical model, the house may be seen as a favorable life setting with a structure and program flexible enough to enable transfer from the therapeutic situation. In actual practice there is no clear dichotomy. The majority of houses seem closer to the traditional medical model. But even these find themselves involved in some socioenvironmental modifications relevant to their residents' problems.

The halfway house is commonly seen as a transitional facility. But the diversity presented by the actual examples points to less recognized functions which deviate considerably from this commonly accepted notion of transition. Again, a bipolar conceptualization is possible. On the one hand, the halfway house may serve a preventive function, substituting entirely for temporary hospitalization. On the other hand, it may serve a supportive function for those who may never be able to live wholly independently.

The data indicate that even with "normal" inmates excluded, ten per cent of the residents of halfway houses have never been hospitalized. For this small group, the concept of transition between hospital and community may be irrelevant. Presumably, these people are in halfway houses as a way of avoiding hospitalization. The halfway house enables them to have a life within the community, but temporarily removed from living situations which might aggravate their problems. In a halfway house they find some measure of support in an environment which, if not actually beneficial, is at least unharmful. They may thus avoid the necessity of breaking off meaningful connections with work, friends, and hobbies, all of which would have to be reestablished if the resident were forced to spend some time in a distant hospital. The halfway house can thus serve as a temporary retreat, enabling a partial moratorium. Such a preventive function can be particularly useful for adolescents, but it also can be useful for others.[1] Halfway houses sometimes think of their work as preventive—according to the public health concept of tertiary prevention—in that they aim to reduce the need for hospital readmission. The potential in providing a way to avoid hospitalization—secondary prevention in a public health sense—is not currently emphasized by halfway houses. The data suggest, however, that prevention in this broader sense may be a possible major function of halfway houses in the future.

At the opposite pole is the resident who has spent considerable time at the hospital and at the halfway house, but is incapable of making the final break and becoming independent. He tends to regard the house as a permanent home. For staff members this "hard-core" person represents an unsolved problem, especially acute when there is any constant proportion of such cases and the house inevitably fills up with permanent residents. Yet there is no inherent logic in the notion that the halfway house must serve as a way station for all. There is a need for houses which serve an "in-between" rather than a transitional function. Undoubtedly, there are many who do not require the total surveillance of hospital life, but who are unable to tolerate the complexities of usual styles of independent living. With the social supports provided by halfway houses, many of these people could become a part of the social community. It may be, then, that certain houses can come to be devoted principally to these people now designated as "hard-core."

---

[1] For example, Fountain House's recent use of its apartments in conjunction with a program of part-time child care to serve mothers with small children. though presently confined to ex-hospitalized women, points to a further preventive potentiality (Fountain House Progress Report, 1965).

Implications

Let us turn from these issues to look at the halfway house in a broader context. Where does the halfway house fit into a general scheme of services for the mentally disturbed? Is it simply an alternative after-care service, along with the day-hospital, the night-hospital, the sheltered workshop? Is it but another way-station on the mythical pilgrimage between sickness in the mental hospital and the holy grail of mental health in the community? Or does what we have discussed in previous chapters imply more for the future than is suggested by these views?

An outgrowth of work of the Joint Commission on Mental Illness and Health was the passage in 1963 by the Congress of the United States of a bill authorizing the establishment of "comprehensive community mental health centers." The bill aims to return the problems of mental disorders to the community. For the large mental hospital, distant and socially alienated from the community, the Act seeks to substitute the concept of an integrated center with an array of services embedded in the community. The center is conceived of not as a physical unit with a single locus but rather as an organized collation of activities, ranging from direct care of the severely disturbed to providing community resources with aids which will enable them to spot and deal with psychological difficulties at early stages.

In order to qualify for Federal funds, the comprehensive community mental health center must provide five "essential" services. These include: (*a*) inpatient care facilities; (*b*) outpatient facilities for adults, children, and families; (*c*) facilities for partial hospitalization, such as day-care centers; (*d*) arrangements for 24-hour emergency care; (*e*) consultation and educational services to community agencies. Also encouraged within the program of the comprehensive center are: (*a*) diagnostic services; (*b*) rehabilitative services, including both social and vocational rehabilitation; (*c*) pre-care and after-care arrangements for those needing hospitalization; (*d*) programs for training of mental health personnel; and (*e*) programs of research and evaluation.

As noted in an official position paper of the American Psychological Association (Smith & Hobbs, 1966), the comprehensive community mental health center represents a fundamental conceptual shift in dealing with mental disorder:

> . . . mental disorder is not the private misery of an individual; it often grows out of and usually contributes to the breakdown of normal sources of social support and understanding, especially the family. It is not just an individual who has faltered; the social systems in which he is embedded through family, school, or job, through religious affiliation or through friendship, have failed to sustain him as an effective participant.
>
> From this view of mental disorder as rooted in the social systems in which the troubled person participates, it follows that the objective of the center staff should be to help the various social systems of which the community is composed to function in ways that develop and sustain the effectiveness of the individuals who take part in them, and to help these community systems regroup their forces to support the person who runs into trouble (p. 500).

The position paper by Smith and Hobbs expresses concern, however, that emphasis on the five "essential" services outlined in the Community Mental Health Center Act, with their focus on the medically traditional inpatient–outpatient core, may negate the potential of new conceptions and their implications for dealing with mental health problems:

> . . . Partial hospitalization and emergency care represent highly desirable, indeed essential, extensions of the traditional clinical services in the direction of greater flexibility and less disruption in patterns of living. Yet the newer approach to community mental health through the social systems in which people are embedded (family, school, neighborhood, factory, etc.) has further implications. For the disturbed person, the goal of community mental health programs should be to help him and the social systems of which he is a member to function together as harmoniously and productively as possible. Such a goal is more practical, and more readily specified, than the elusive concept of "cure," which misses the point that for much mental disorder the trouble lies not within the skin of the

individual but in the interpersonal systems through which he is related to others (p. 501).

Smith and Hobbs emphasize that this conceptualization implies centers should not be simply programs imposed onto communities by mental health professionals; they suggest that community involvement and community control are essential, and that communities may be better served by gaining greater perspective on what is essential. Thus they comment that facilities and services must be conceived in relation to particular needs and that these needs for a particular community may involve schools, courts, churches, business and industry, labor groups, social and welfare agencies. They note the traditional barriers and cross-purposes that so often separate mental health services from other agencies serving the community, and they suggest that if there is to be continuity of services for the disturbed there must be communication and freedom of movement not only between specifically labeled mental health agencies but also among all systems of the community. Problem groups they note as particularly neglected and particularly in need of innovative approaches involving broad community focus are the seriously disturbed, the poor and disadvantaged, and children and youth. Their final recommendation emphasizes the importance of planning for flexibility and for adaptation to social change.

In this context, let us return to our consideration of halfway houses. In the Community Mental Health Center Act they receive along with home visiting and foster-care arrangements a secondary mention as part of—not "essential" but recommended—after-care services. Yet, as we have seen, halfway houses, in their diversity, represent more than after-care with its connotations of medical recuperation for ex-hospital patients. We have seen that the populations of halfway houses range from those who have never been hospitalized at all, through those who have been out of hospitals for some years before coming to a halfway house, to those who arrive after ten or more years incarceration in hospital back wards. We have seen houses which choose only those residents who have high potential for rehabilitation; but we have seen other houses concentrating on "high-risk" residents. Moreover, we have noted the emphasis in some houses on short, limited stays for residents and the contrasting acceptance by other houses of semipermanent residence. Our descriptions of the functions that halfway houses undertake illustrate a similar diversity and an astonishing range of activities. Tasks of socialization—from handling ordinary daily routines of living to management of complex social relations, tasks of vocational help and work orientation, tasks of psychotherapy—of personal and interpersonal change: all are part—some houses emphasizing one aspect, some another—of what halfway houses do. Given the diversity and the array of activities with which we have become familiar in previous chapters, where, then, do halfway houses fit?

Traditionally, approaches to psychological change have taken either of two directions. One has been to focus on the person, arguing that through effecting change in the person we alter his approach to and relations with his environment. Mastery of the environment, within the range of possibilities it offers, is seen, in a sense, as an epiphenomenon of successful personal change. The alternative direction has been to focus on the environment. The argument here is that by effecting environmental changes we can alter personal stresses and increase opportunities for successful experiences. The development of personal strengths can be seen, in a sense, as an outgrowth of appropriately gauged environmental changes.

The balance of opinion favoring one of these approaches over the other has no doubt varied with the temper of the times, and at any given time with personal predilections. Moreover, attempts at rational dialogue between the two are apt to be confounded by yet another version of the mind-body problem—the problem of personality and environment. There are, nonetheless, bases for pragmatic decisions between approaches. For example, for the middle- or upper-class neurotic, whose environment offers choices among manifold opportunities, and who himself seems in good control of his environment—except, of course, where it impinges on neurotic problems—a program of environmental changes would seem to offer little prospect of permanent success. Change here would seem to require a focus on psychic rather than environmental factors. Psychoanalytic theory, in its discussion of the dynamics of anxiety and defense and in its elaborations on psychopathology, tells us why this should be so. If, on the other hand, we are dealing with the psychological problems of those who are socially and economically disadvantaged, it would seem reasonable to attempt to improve environments so they can offer opportunities for psychological growth. Freud once noted that one could not psychoanalyze a man who was physically hungry, implying that the press of severe reality problems precludes an atmosphere favorable to psychic exploration. Indeed, as Robert Reiff (1966) suggests, a sense of self-determination—the notion that one can play a role in determining what happens to him—must precede any interest in self-actualization. For the disadvantaged, then, we must create situations—that is, environments—in which people can affect their circumstances to as to broaden opportunities for change.

Though these concepts focus on change, there is another dimension we need to consider. Whether the emphasis is on the person or on the environment, goals can vary. What will the change accomplish? In Chapter 2 we noted Rapaport's (1960) comments on confusions between designs appropriate to treatment, "the reorganization of individual dynamics," and those appropriate to rehabilitation, "the adjustment of the individual to his social role." Similar distinctions are implied throughout the literature, but are seldom made explicit. Thus, the term "therapy" is used loosely, sometimes referring to goals of socialization, sometimes referring to goals of personal integration. Another way, then, of studying this dimension is by considering a range of approaches from educative to integrative. Educative approaches can focus on the individual person—as in providing information, inculcating skills, or fostering different behaviors or motives through support or appropriate reinforcement; they can, on the other hand, focus on the environment through, for example, employer or parent education, or through ecological changes which provide new opportunities for learning. Integrative approaches concentrating on the person are well known—their emphasis is on reorganization, reconstruction, insight, individuation, self-realization; integrative approaches via an environmental orientation are more obscure—they seem to be illustrated in some expressive methods, in some specialized approaches to living—as in some forms of monastic training—or in psychological "brainwashing," and perhaps, too, under some drug conditions.

Our discussions indicate that halfway houses differ on where they choose to put their emphases. For many the weight is on person—and integration-directed change, either through therapy programs within the house or through emphases on outside psychotherapy—the house sometimes being seen as a "holding operation" for allowing the "real" work of psychotherapy to go on. For some the focus is on direct education, using the tasks of daily living to provide opportunities for socialization. A few houses—of which Wellmet is the most explicit—seem to concentrate on opportunities for varying the social environment of the house to induce favorable learning experiences. And a few others—notably some rural houses—strive through their work programs to create environments which are directed not so much toward goals of socialization but toward promoting a sense of personal wholeness and integration.

Yet though each house may be *somewhat* specialized in its orientation, with a primary focus on one aspect rather than another, no house seems completely limited to a single approach. There is not only diversity among houses, but also within any house a variety of functions and activities. Any aspect of living at any house can—and probably does at some time—come into a focus of attention. How to sew a hem, how to get a job, how to get along with a roommate, or how to think about life are all relevant problems in a halfway house.

The halfway house, unlike the mental hospital, is not a "total institution," any more than the family is. Its controls on residents are limited and residents are encouraged to have lives outside the house. Its approach to problems is not monolithic. Residents are socialized to house rules, but they may also play a part in changing those rules. Residents are, in a sense, at times patients in the house, but at other times working colleagues, helpers, friends, tenants, and apprentices. Inconsistencies can be seen not as breaches in an impenetrable wall of authority but as individual issues which can be worked out as parts of life. The small number of people, the relative lack of hierarchical structure, the intimacy of arrangements, all enhance flexibility in approaching problems. As needs arise staff can shift rapidly from focus on the house as a whole to focus on an individual, or from focus on problems of socialization to focus on problems of personal integration.

The activities of the halfway house thus cover a broad front. In its breadth of activities the halfway house is similar to the mental hospital. But it more closely resembles the child residential institution which must be concerned not only with problems of personality change but also with growth and development and with education and socialization. The diversity and breadth of functions of the halfway house have a similar rationale. Most residents are labeled as schizophrenic. The label provides us with no answers, but it does tell us that the problems of those who carry it are—in most though perhaps not all cases—not specific and not localized. It tells us of massive disturbance—in socialization, in interpersonal relations and object attachments, in identificatory images, in perception, thought, affect and will. Long incarceration adds to this. No single technique or method of approach can be capable of dealing with this array of issues. Were a pill eliminating the bizarre dramatic symptoms of schizophrenia discovered, we would still have, in most cases, to deal with the issues which confront the ex-schizophrenic as he tries to establish a fuller life.

In the hospital the patient is acculturated to a single role —that of hospital patient. The process of acculturation to this role, the career lines which follow, and the effects of the process have been vividly described by sociologists and social anthropologists, and there is a growing awareness of the penalties exacted by hospitalization. In contrast, the halfway house acculturates its residents to no single role. Erikson, Sharp, & Maeda (1963), in an unpublished analysis of interactions between staff and residents of Woodley House, emphasize this point. They note that not only is there no single role appropriate to a halfway house resident, but also that the house provides the opportunity for testing out any of a variety of roles in a situation that is relatively benign and tolerant. That a similar ambiguity exists in relation to staff is suggested by the variety of occupational backgrounds found among halfway house directors. Whatever his background, the staff person carries multiple roles in the halfway house. That this creates a unique position is suggested by Landy and Greenblatt (1965):

> Some of the women view Miss Grant as an understanding social worker, and feel that is her reason for being in the House. Miss Grant does not think the women give her a title: "I think the girls are a little suspicious of titles; doctors and social workers *do* things to them or they suspect an ulterior motive." She was asked if she had a title. "No, as far as I know I'm just Miss Grant—just someone to talk with and not someone who is going to change their lives." However, the observer felt that she does to an extent change the lives of these women. She seemed deeply committed to "trying to help [the residents] toward a better understanding of daily living and their part in it" (pp. 26–27).

The halfway house thus provides its member with a moratorium not in the sense of a divorcement from life but in the sense of providing an arena in which, unlike other arenas, the major task is that of testing out the various aspects of oneself. Ideally, then, before leaving the house the resident has made a beginning in finding himself and his stance in relation to others.

Morris and Charlotte Schwartz (1964) in a volume which represents the final report of the Project on Patterns of Patient Care—one of ten study groups established by the Joint Commission on Mental Illness and Health—note that ex-patients' avoidance of after-care represents a rejection of the stigmatized patient status. The ex-patient who avoids after-care, who tries to "pass," may, they suggest, be trying to divest himself of a deviant label so as to avoid permanent alienation from society (pp. 283–285). In discussing the need for "normal" social roles for ex-patients and the need for change in community response, the Schwartzes comment:

Many practitioners take the stand that they are only seeking for the ex-mental-hospital patient the same status as that accorded physically ill persons. But it is clear that they want more for ex-patients than the mere exemption from responsibilities that are allowed by the sick role. What they are asking is that society develop another status for ex-patients, one that will help them *learn how to live* in society' while at the same time *not penalize them for their failures* to perform adequately during the learning period. Thus, what the practitioner wants is not that the ex-patient be dealt with by society as a sick person but as a *trainee in living.* This is a vastly different matter and involves not only the acceptance of an ex-patient's inability to function but also his right to experiment in society with finding more satisfactory ways of living. If and when such a role becomes established, it will symbolize a basic alteration in the way mental illness is conceived in our society and a profound change in the way it is handled by laymen and practitioners (italics all the Schwartzes, pp. 287–288).

For the ex-patient, then, our data all suggest that the halfway house provides the opportunities for training in living. But we can go a step further than this. In discussing recommendations for changes in in-patient hospital treatment Schwartz and Schwartz (1964) say:

Two changes will have to be made. The first is the revision of the role of the patient. Genuine respect for the patient and for the dignity of his person, some privacy in living arrangements, and opportunities for the cultivation of self-esteem must be built into his role. In addition, his responsibility and share in decisions may be increased; opportunities must be provided for work and constructive activity that approximate normal living; and normal social performance, consistent with his sociocultural background, family context, and reference groups should be made possible. What is needed for the patient is a role that primarily serves his interests and is oriented toward his improvement and not toward the staff's convenience or the institution's conventions.

The second change calls for a restructuring to make all levels of staff agents of, and vehicles for, the patient's therapeutic resocialization. Staff members would support and facilitate the patient's role as described above. This means that, through participation with patients, they would encourage the optimum amount of responsibility and independence in decision making of which each is capable. Further, they would use their interpersonal relations with patients as instruments to teach them, directly and indirectly, how to live according to accepted norms and would advise them in their attempts to understand and successfully negotiate difficult and painful human experiences. Finally, they would bring about social situations and group contexts in which patients would have opportunities for learning new modes of human relations (p. 300).

Such changes require mechanisms for insuring institutional flexibility:

If flexibility of response to patients' changing needs is to be achieved in the mental hospital, there must be a change in the size of the hospital and of individual wards. Large mental hospitals are notoriously cumbersome, slow in responding to patients' needs, and difficult to free from their rigidities. But in smaller hospitals with fewer patients on a ward as well as increased staff-patient ratios, the staff can focus on patients as individuals, and at the same time the small numbers of patients can live together in ways that resemble life outside the institution (Schwartz & Schwartz, 1964, p. 301).

Application of the principle of diversification to a particular inpatient treatment institution might lead to the creation of a variety of relatively independent subunits within which its various patients are cared for and treated. Or a number of independent treatment units, each based on a different institutional model, might comprise the diversified facilities of a community or region. Thus, in addition to the conventional model of the mental hospital with its range of treatment modalities, other institutions might be introduced. One, modeled on the home, might be composed of a group of small cottages with from eight to twelve "patient-members," run by a male and female "staff member," in which the primary emphasis is on family living and on interpersonal processes of resocialization. Another model might copy Gheel in Belgium, in which the families of an entire community provide the resocialization experience by accepting patients into their homes to live with them as members of the family. Others might be modeled on the school, focusing on teaching social and other skills in a manner approximating, but not duplicating, that of an ordinary classroom. Finally, still others might be modeled on a factory or workshop where the patient learns work habits and skills and is remunerated for work performance. All models might profitably be experimented with and used in various combinations to establish diversity in help. This might lead to the development of a treatment setting better adapted to patients' needs than any we now have (Schwartz & Schwartz, 1964, pp. 301–302).

Prospects

Although in their suggestions the Schwartzes continue to speak within the framework of mental hospital reform, it is important to note that the models they propose extend far outside this framework. As we noted in Chapter 2 and elsewhere in this book, there have been periodic, intensive and dramatic efforts to reform the mental hospital. In the long run these efforts have borne sparse fruit. It is easy to attribute the lack of success to inadequate funds or to unavailability of professionally trained personnel, and certainly these lacks are part of the story. But the causes of failure in reforms are also—as Schwartz and Schwartz suggest (pp. 82–83) —embedded in the social structure. We have in earlier chapters noted how hospital structure predisposes toward particular functional arrangements and particular social relationships. Attempts at reform must inevitably fail when they are grafted onto a structure that is inappropriate to them.

If we follow out the suggestions made by Schwartz and Schwartz, we shall not be merely reforming the mental hospital. The models they suggest for dealing with mental disturbance are not extensions of hospital treatment. Rather we are adopting here a new mode of thinking about mental disturbance.

We would suggest then that the halfway house is not simply an auxiliary after-care service for the mental hospital. We would suggest rather that a potential network of halfway, three-quarter way, and quarter-way houses represents an alternative to the mental hospital. And we would suggest that a network of such houses, with opportunities for mobility among them, offers a more appropriate structure and far greater opportunities for rehabilitation and re-integration than does the mental hospital. The diverse models presented in our studies offer possibilities for a range of social settings gauged to a range of psychological disturbance—from the adolescent who needs a temporary relief from the intensity of his family life to the schizophrenic whose massive and diffuse psychopathology requires him to have help in all aspects of living. It would be wrong, however, to think of the halfway house as a smaller, or more humane, or more individualized, or more efficient mental hospital; it would be wrong to think of it as requiring fewer resources than the hospital. It is not a hospital at all. It provides arrangements for living through a structure designed to make daily experiences useful rather than harmful. But equally important is its service as liaison between the resident and community resources. Unlike the hospital which gathers all resources under its wings—and whose size is in part related to this—it is important that the halfway house *is* limited. Because of its limitations the halfway house must call upon the resources of its members and of the surrounding community. For a halfway house to function properly it needs to find and work with its community, by which we mean not the local neighborhood but that community which consists of shops and services, of employers and job opportunities, of psychotherapists and clinics, of recreational and social facilities. The halfway house cannot stand alone and the usefulness of its transactions with its residents is based on the fact that it does not stand alone. Neither it nor its residents can be isolated from the community.

The halfway house needs the hospital. Hospitals are traditionally specialized emergency facilities capable of providing care, security, and technical competence in cases of physical or physiological crises. Some equivalent is needed for psychological crises. It is likely that many who are mentally disturbed will suffer at some time or another disruptions which are so acute as to demand the total protection which hospitals can provide. If hospitals were freed from responsibility for long-term incarceration and if hospital staff and patients were freed from the stigma which comes from this function, crisis episodes might be dealt with far more effectively. Intensive emergency short-term service, responsive flexibly to need, could be part of urban general hospital facilities. Professional resources could be maximized for intensive professional work. There would be a dignity and an excitement to such work not presently found in hospital practice.

On the other side, we have seen that the transitional function of the halfway house does not end sharply when the resident moves from the house. At some houses former residents may for a time continue to board or spend some evening time at the house or they may return for occasional visits. This, too, has a rationale. Transition needs to be seen not as discrete, discontinuous segments but as a series of graduated steps. Clinics and social agencies, joint living arrangements with minimal or no supervision, ex-patient clubs can all be useful in providing and extending these directions.

If the halfway house does not and cannot stand alone, the implication is that it cannot be evaluated in isolation. If we have neglected the issue of research in relation to success or failure, it is because an altered conception of mental disturbance and its treatment demands an altered conception of research. If we conceive of change solely in terms of "cure" of a specific disease, then evaluative research will take its present form: the introduction of a specific procedure with measurements taken before and after. If, on the other hand, we conceive of the approach to change in severe psychological disturbance as an attempt to develop and integrate patterns of living where these have suffered major disruption, research must take a different form.

In one sense the latter conception makes research simpler. "Any day out of the hospital is a good day"—as one halfway house director puts it—becomes a legitimate statement. If someone who would otherwise be hospitalized performs a day's work, pays a day's taxes, helps another, something is accomplished—even if the person must later return to the hospital. In another sense systematic research becomes more complicated. For success can no longer be evaluated in relation to a single intervention. Rather, as with development, one must think of a series of steps to be negotiated. Thus, for example, when we are faced with the issues of massive psycho-pathology, psychotherapeutic efforts cannot stand alone. Psycho-therapy will fail if living arrangements prevent its being utilized. Psychotherapy and appropriate living arrangements, in turn, assure no high probability of success if there is a fundamental lack of skill in daily routine aspects of living. A further choice-point for success or failure involves capacities for getting and holding a job; and negotiating these steps may still be insufficient if ability to estab-lish meaningful social relationships cannot be developed. Should such a view seem needlessly complicated or unpragmatic, we must remind ourselves of studies of animal courtship or maternal be-havior which illustrate the dependence of a final state on a series of sequentially ordered partial accomplishments, and where failure at any one stage disrupts the chances of a successful outcome. Can we then demand that the process of overcoming massive psycho-logical disturbance be any simpler or that studying the process require less sophistication?

Even given a dramatic biochemical discovery which elimi-nates some of the phenomena of severe disturbance, the issues of how to live with oneself and with others will continue to be basic for those who have suffered massive disruption in living. Halfway houses are laboratories for dealing with these issues and they can also serve to investigate what conditions are necessary and sufficient to allow these sufferers to establish a life in the social community.

Halfway houses will, we predict, continue to increase.[2] They offer professional staff a degree of freedom and autonomy that does not exist in hospitals. Interest and motivation can be maximized. Administrative simplicity enables flexibility and ex-perimentation. Nor does staff suffer from the enclosedness and iso-lation that develop in total institutions. The opportunities halfway houses offer for training and for careers have not yet been fully used.

For their development halfway houses need stable finan-cial support. Perhaps some houses can manage independently,

---

[2] A casual estimate indicates that there are, as of this writing in mid-1967, more than 100 halfway houses in the United States.

though even these require initial help. More important is that if halfway houses have to be supported by their resident populations, many of those who most need their services would be denied. As we have suggested, halfway houses also need support from and integration with other institutional services. We have implied that a network of communication and interchange of ideas and even of residents could improve the work of halfway houses. Furthermore, if the movement grows, issues of professional standards and qualifications will arise.

Each of these developments suggests an increased institutionalization of the halfway house movement. And if halfway houses follow the course of other institutional developments they will almost inevitably be pushed toward organization. Halfway house directors are resistant to an organized association. The resistance is based not only on personal predilections for independence, but also on an awareness that the strength of the halfway house movement derives in part from diversity and lack of standardization and from freedom to diverge from traditional psychiatric models. Most halfway houses do not yet clearly recognize the extent of innovation they represent. The test for the future will be in meeting problems of organization and support without losing the impetus and excitement generated by the new concepts and new hopes they offer.

APPENDIX A

HALFWAY HOUSE
QUESTIONNAIRE

(Letter accompanying questionnaire)

In the last few years Halfway Houses have mushroomed all over the country. Woodley House, established in the District of Columbia in 1959, one of these. As part of the Woodley House Research program, being conducted under a National Institute of Mental Health grant, we are making comprehensive study of existing Halfway House facilities. Presently we know of about 50 such houses.

The accompanying questionnaire is designed to provide a great deal information about Halfway Houses and make it available to us all. I hope that you will be able to complete the questionnaire fully and return it, along with your brochure if you have one. Where any question is already answered your brochure, just note this in the appropriate place. If there are any questions you wish to discuss more fully, please feel free to continue on last page or to add additional pages.

Upon completion of the study, all respondents will receive a resume of the findings or a reprint of a published article. Rules of confidentiality will, of course, be respected. We would appreciate your notifying us of other Halfway Houses in your area to whom this questionnaire should be sent to sure the completeness of our data.

Thank you so much,

ORIGINS AND POPULATION

1. When was the Halfway House established? _____

2. By whom: Name of person or institution _____

   With sponsor (GIVE NAME) _____

   Unsponsored

3. Is it intended as a profit-making operation?   ☐ No   ☐ Yes

4. With what purpose did this House originate? _____

   _____

   _____

   _____

5. Was there a particular group or groups for which the house was intended?   ☐ No   ☐ Yes

   If yes, what was the group? _____

   5a. In practice has it worked out that the House is serving this group?   ☐ No   ☐ Yes

   5b. If no, please indicate how the actual group has differed? _____

   _____

6. Was there a decision at the outset that a particular group or groups could not be served?

                                                                  ☐ No   ☐ Yes

   6a. If yes, what group or groups were these? _____

   _____

   6b. Are they still excluded?   ☐ No   ☐ Yes

   6c. If no, has experience led you to exclude any group or groups?   ☐ No   ☐ Yes

   6d. If yes, what was the group, and what actually happened that led you to make that decision?

   _____

   _____

   _____

7. What are the most frequent psychiatric diagnoses among the residents? _____

   _____

8. If there were original requirements for selection of residents, what were they? _____

   _____

9. Do present requirements differ from these?   ☐ No   ☐ Yes

    If yes, how do they differ? _____

    _____

10. Does the house prefer to select:

    Residents who resemble one another diagnostically or symptomatically.   ☐

    Residents who differ from one another diagnostically or symptomatically.   ☐

    This factor does not influence selection.   ☐

11. How many residents are there at present? _____ Is this:

                                            ☐ Average
                                            ☐ More
                                            ☐ Fewer

12. Of your present residents, how many are . . . (PLEASE FILL IN NUMBER)

                                    Male   Female

                        _____ 20 or younger   _____ 20 or younger
                        _____ 21 to 40   _____ 21 to 40
                        _____ 41 to 65   _____ 41 to 65
                        _____ 65 and over   _____ 65 and over

13. Of your present residents, how many . . . . . (PLEASE FILL IN NUMBER)

    _____ have never been hospitalized

    _____ came at discharge or while still on books of a mental hospital

    _____ were out of the hospital one to five years before coming

    _____ other, please explain _____

    _____

14. Of your present residents, how many were referred by . . . . . (GIVE NUMBER)

    _____ hospitals

    _____ social agencies

    _____ private psychiatrists, social workers or psychologists

    _____ other, please explain _____

15. Does the prospective resident visit the house and discuss his coming with a staff member?

                                            ☐ Usually
                                            ☐ Sometimes
                                            ☐ Never

16. Is there a continuing contact between the referral source and the house?

                                            ☐ Usually
                                            ☐ Sometimes
                                            ☐ Never

17. Does the house have legal responsibility for any of its residents?   ☐ No   ☐ Yes

If yes, about how many out of the present group? _____

STAFF

18. Who is on the staff of the house?

Job Title	Academic/Professional Training if any	Years of Experience	Number Hours/Week

19. Do any staff members wear uniforms on duty? Star (*) them above.

20. Who is responsible for making the day-to-day administrative decisions? _____

_____

21. Who is responsible for making the policy decisions? _____

_____

22. Is there at least one staff member on duty at all times?   ☐ No   ☐ Yes

23. Are there any arrangements for supervision of staff? If there are, would you describe them briefly?

_____

_____

24. Have you had staffing problems, either relating to quality of staff available or rate of turnover?

     ☐ No   ☐ Yes

24a. If yes, could you discuss these briefly? _____

_____

_____

_____

PHYSICAL PLANT

25. What is the area adjacent to the Halfway House?

☐ Hospital grounds
☐ Urban-commercial area
☐ Urban-residential area
☐ Suburban area
☐ Rural area

26. Did the Halfway House start with an already acquired building?

☐ No   ☐ Yes
go to (d)

26a. If yes, please describe the building (age, size structural type) _____

_____

26b. How satisfactory is it?   ☐ Very   ☐ Somewhat   ☐ Unsatisfactory

26c. What, if any, changes would you like to see made? _____

_____

26d. If no, what did you look for as an ideal accommodation? _____

_____

26e. What did you get? (Describe age, size, structural type) _____

_____

26f. How satisfactory is it?   ☐ Very   ☐ Somewhat   ☐ Unsatisfactory

26g. What, if any, changes would you like to see made? _____

_____

27. If there are bedrooms, how many are there? _____

28. If dormitories, what is the number, and bed capacity of each? _____

_____

29. How many other rooms are there in general use? _____

30. Are any rooms closed to residents?

☐ No   ☐ Yes

If yes, which are these? _____

31. What recreational facilities does the House have? _____

_____

_____

_____

_____

RULES

32. Does the House have written rules?   ☐ No   ☐ Yes

    If <u>yes</u>, please append a copy or summarize below.

33. Does the House have unwritten but understood rules?   ☐ No   ☐ Yes

    If <u>yes</u>, please summarize in space below.

Description of Rules (Please include all rules dealing with noise, hours, visitors, smoking and drinking, use of various rooms, leaves and absences and others. If both written and unwritten rules are included, differentiate them) PUT A STAR (*) BY FREQUENTLY BROKEN RULES AND A CHECK BY MOST NECESSARY ONES.

_____

_____

_____

_____

_____

_____

_____

_____

_____

_____

_____

_____

34. Have any rules been dropped, changed or added?   ☐ No   ☐ Yes

    If <u>yes</u>, which were these and what were the changes? _____

    _____

    _____

35. What techniques of enforcement are used? Please describe them and comment on their effectiveness?

    _____

    _____

FINANCIAL ARRANGEMENTS

36. When the house was begun, what was the principal source of funds? _____

    _____

37. Were there any conditions to be met in order to receive this support?   ☐ No   ☐ Yes

    37a. If <u>yes</u>, what were they? _____

    _____

    _____

    37b. Is this arrangement still in effect?   ☐ No   ☐ Yes

37c. If <u>no</u>, what is the present arrangement? _____

---

38. Do people in the House pay fees?   ☐ No   ☐ Yes

If <u>no</u>, please turn to next section on <u>Work and Jobs</u>

   38a. If <u>yes</u>, is it a set fee or does it differ for individuals?

      ☐ Set. If set, what is it? $ _____ per month.

      ☐ Differs. If differs, what is the range? $ _____ to $ _____ per month.

   38b. How is the amount determined? (Be specific, for example: $100/mo. for the poorest to $400 mo. wealthiest)

---

39. What proportion of total operating expense is covered by fees?   ☐ 0 – 24%
                                                                     ☐ 25 – 49%
                                                                     ☐ 50 – 74%
                                                                     ☐ 75% or more

40. Do you think the present fees are adequate?   ☐ No   ☐ Yes

   If <u>no</u>, are you planning to increase them?   ☐ No   ☐ Yes

41. Have you had any difficulty about setting or collecting fees?   ☐ No   ☐ Yes

   If <u>yes</u>, please describe the problems. _____

WORK AND JOBS

42. Aside from paying fees, do people who live in the house contribute work which would otherwise require staff or hired labor?

                                                 ☐ No   ☐ Yes

   If <u>yes</u>, is it ☐ formally assigned

               ☐ informal and at the resident's own initiative

               ☐ other, please explain. _____

43. Do any of the residents hold paying jobs outside the House?   ☐ No   ☐ Yes

   If <u>no</u>, please skip to question 45.

   If <u>yes</u>, how many presently hold paying jobs? _____

   What kinds of jobs are these? _____

   Who arranges them? _____

Who takes responsibility for the income from them? _____

Are there any special arrangements or concessions for jobholders?   ☐ No   ☐ Yes

If yes, what are these? _____

44. Is holding a job outside of the house encouraged by staff?   ☐ No   ☐ Yes

45. Do any of the residents do volunteer work on a regular basis?   ☐ No   ˙☐ Yes

THERAPY

46. Was it planned to provide therapy in the House?   ☐ No   ☐ Yes
                                                                           go to (e)

If yes, describe your therapy program (including psychotherapy, group therapy, chemotherapy and any other forms of therapy used, and an approximate number of the resident population involved in each type).

_____

_____

_____

_____

_____

46b. Are you satisfied with the therapy program(s) as presently arranged?   ☐ No   ☐ Yes

46c. If no, what changes would you like to see made? _____

_____

_____

46d. If changes have been made since the beginning, what were the problems that caused the changes to

come about? _____

_____

_____

46e. If no, were any provisions made to have therapy provided outside the House?   ☐ No   ☐ Yes

If no, skip to the section on Discharge.

If yes, was this set as a condition of residence?   ☐ No   ☐ Yes

46f. Have there been difficulties between the house and outside therapists?   ☐ No   ☐ Yes

If yes, briefly describe the areas of problems. _____

_____

_____

46g. Who pays the therapist's fees? _____ _____

46h. Are there periodic consultations with the therapists? ☐ No ☐ Yes

    If yes, are these: ☐ Formal and at regular intervals or

                         ☐ Informal according to need

46i. What disciplines are represented among the therapists? _____

_____

DISCHARGE

47. The average length of stay of a resident is? _____

48. Who decides when a resident is ready for discharge? _____

49. Do any residents stay quite indefinitely at the House? ☐ No ☐ Yes

50. Where do residents go when they leave the House?. About what percentage:

                                 %

             _____ return to the hospital within the first year

             _____ return to their families

             _____ go into a foster home situation

             _____ live independently in the community

             _____ other (please specify) _____

                           _____

51. Are residents encouraged to come back to visit after they leave? ☐ No ☐ Yes

    If yes, do they? ☐ No ☐ Yes

52. Is there any follow-up of residents after they leave? ☐ No ☐ Yes

    If yes, please describe briefly. _____

_____

_____

COMMUNITY RELATIONS

53. When the Halfway House was begun, was there opposition from the community? ☐ No ☐ Yes

    If yes, please describe the type of opposition and ways in which you dealt with it. _____

_____

_____

    Have the problems been satisfactorily resolved at this time? ☐ No ☐ Yes

    If no, have you any hopes or plans for working out a solution? ☐ No ☐ Yes

54. In general, how do you think the community views the House?

    ☐ they have a feeling of interest and concern

    ☐ as a place for "recovered" mental patients, therefore safe, o.k.

    ☐ bitterly, that it reduces the property values in the area

    ☐ fearfully, that it may cause unpleasant or dangerous incidents

    ☐ neutrally, or without knowledge or interest

    ☐ community attitude is not known

55. Are any community facilities used by the residents of the House?   ☐ No   ☐ Yes

If **yes**, please list those frequently used. Include social agencies, employment agencies, educational and recreational facilities. _____

_____

_____

_____

56. Is movement into the community actively encouraged by the staff?   ☐ No   ☐ Yes

If **yes**, what means are used? _____

_____

57. In conclusion, is there anything unique or especially effective about this House that you would like other people in the field to know about? Would you describe it? _____

_____

_____

_____

_____

_____

_____

_____

_____

_____

_____

_____

APPENDIX B

HALFWAY HOUSES IN THE STUDY

Non-VA-Affiliated Houses

CALIFORNIA

Conard House
2441 Jackson Street
San Francisco, California
Capacity: 28

Harvey House
1835 Middlefield Road
Palo Alto, California
Capacity: 10

Portals
2 Houses: 1615 South Street, Andrews
            Place
        Los Angeles, California
        Capacity: 10 men

        3974 Ingraham Street
        Los Angeles, California
        Capacity: 9 women

Quarters
854 Jackson Street
Santa Clara, California
2 Houses: 7 men
            7 women

DISTRICT OF COLUMBIA

Woodley House
2711 Connecticut Avenue
Washington, D.C.
Capacity: 10

IOWA

River Heights House
1511 So. Division Street
Sioux City, Iowa
Capacity: 25

KANSAS

Meadowlark Homestead
Newton, Kansas
Capacity: 30

KENTÚCKY

Stepping Stone
Lexington, Kentucky
Capacity: 9 women

Colonial Inn
Louisville, Kentucky
Capacity: 9 women

MARYLAND

1 Lawrence Court
Rockville, Maryland
Capacity: 20

MASSACHUSETTS

Gould Farm
Great Barrington, Massachusetts
Capacity: 25

Rutland Corner House
1027 Beacon Street
Brookline, Massachusetts

Wellmet
11 Marie Street
Cambridge, Massachusetts
Capacity: 5

MICHIGAN

Mary Hulbert House
Lafayette Clinic
951 E. Lafayette Street
Detroit, Michigan
Capacity: 10 girls—ages 17–25

MISSOURI

Rehabilitation House
St. Louis State Hospital
5400 Arsenal Street
St. Louis, Missouri
Capacity: 9

NEW HAMPSHIRE

Crossroads
Orford, New Hampshire
Capacity: 4

NEW YORK

Fountain House
412 West 47th Street
New York City, New York
Capacity: 24

OREGON

Gutman House
427 Southwest 11th Avenue
Portland, Oregon
Capacity: 12

WEST VIRGINIA

Rehabilitation House for Men
538 Adams Avenue
Huntington, West Virginia
Capacity: 12 men

TEXAS

Mental Health Association of Bexar
    County
117 Avenue A.
San Antonio, Texas
Capacity: 14

Rehabilitation House for Women
406 Fifth Avenue
Huntington, West Virginia
Capacity: 12 women

VA-Affiliated Houses

UTAH

Alpine House
138 So. 3rd West
Provo, Utah
Capacity: 16

ARKANSAS

Little Rock VA Hospital
North Little Rock, Arkansas
2 Houses: 21 men (total)

COLORADO

VERMONT

Rehabilitation Houses
2 Houses: Montpelier, Vermont
    Capacity: 12
    Burlington, Vermont
    Capacity: 12

Fort Lyon VA Hospital
Fort Lyon, Colorado
Capacity: 24 men

KENTUCKY

Spring Lake Ranch
Cuttingsville, Vermont
Capacity: 30

Lexington VA Hospital, Horseshoe
    Lodge
Lexington, Kentucky
Capacity: 40 men

Lexington VA Hospital
Lexington, Kentucky
Capacity: 4 men

MASSACHUSETTS

Foster Home Cottage
Brockton VA Hospital
Brockton, Massachusetts
Capacity: 12 men (on hospital
grounds)

MISSISSIPPI

Gulfport VA Hospital
Gulfport, Mississippi
Capacity: 21 men

NEW YORK

Montrose VA Hospital
Montrose, New York
Capacity: 10 men

NORTH CAROLINA

Salisbury VA Hospital
Salisbury, North Carolina
Capacity: 4 men

OHIO

Chilicothe VA Hospital
Chilicothe, Ohio
Capacity: 4 men

PENNSYLVANIA

Coatsville VA Hospital
Coatsville, Pennsylvania
Capacity: 8 men

TENNESSEE

Murfreesboro VA Hospital
Murfreesboro, Tennessee
Capacity: 7 men

WYOMING

Sheridan VA Hospital
Sheridan, Wyoming
House is in Story, Wyoming (rural)
Capacity: 10 men

*Did not answer questionnaire and not
included in the study; sent brochure*

Edgemont House
4841 Hollywood Boulevard
Los Angeles, California

REFERENCES

Action for mental health. Final report of the Joint Commission on Mental Illness and Health, 1961. New York: Basic Books, 1961.

Appleby, L., Proaño, A., & Perry, R. Theoretical vs. empirical treatment models: an exploratory investigation. In L. Appleby, J. M. Scher, & J. Cumming, *Chronic schizophrenia.* Glencoe, Ill.: Free Press, 1960. Pp. 226–247.

Ayllon, T., & Haughton, E. Control of the behavior of schizophrenic patients by food. *Journal of the Experimental Analysis of Behavior,* 1962, 5, 343–352.

Ayllon, T., & Michael, J. The psychiatric nurse as a behavioral engineer. *Journal of the Experimental Analysis of Behavior,* 1959, 2, 323–334.

Baker, A., Davies, R. L., & Sivadon, P. *Psychiatric services and architecture.* Public Health Papers No. 1. Geneva, Switzerland: World Health Organization, 1959.

Barker, R. G. Ecology and motivation in M. R. Jones (Ed.), *Nebraska symposium on motivation.* Lincoln: University of Nebraska Press, 1960. Pp. 1–49.

Barker, R. G. (Ed.) *The stream of behavior: explorations of its structure and content.* New York: Appleton-Century-Crofts, 1963.

Barker, R. G. Explorations in ecological psychology. *American Psychologist.* 1965, 20, 1–14.

Barker, R. G., & Gump, P. V. *Big school, small school; high school size and student behavior.* Stanford, Calif.: Stanford Univerity Press, 1964.

Bateson, G., Jackson, D. D., Haley, J., & Weakland, J. Toward a theory of schizophrenia. *Behavioral Science,* 1956, 1, 251–264.

227

Bateson, G., Jackson, D. D., Haley, J., & Weakland, J. A note on the double bind—1962. *Family Process*, 1963, 2, 34–51.

Beard, J. H., & Goldman, E. Major problems. *Rehabilitation Record*, 1964, 5 (2), 14–16.

Beard, J. H., Pitt, R. B., Fisher, S. H., & Goertzel, V. Evaluating the effectiveness of a psychiatric rehabilitation program. *American Journal of Orthopsychiatry*, 1963, 33, 701–712.

Beard, J. H., Schmidt, J. R., & Smith, Mary M. The use of transitional employment in the rehabilitation of the psychiatric patient. *Journal of Nervous and Mental Disease*, 1963, 136, 507–514.

Beard, J. H., Schmidt, J. R., Smith, Mary M., & Dincin, J. Three aspects of psychiatric rehabilitation at Fountain House. *Mental Hygiene*, 1964, 48(1), 11–21.

Beers, C. W. *A mind that found itself*. Garden City, N.Y.: Doubleday, 1953.

Bell, D. *Work and it discontents*. Boston: Beacon Press, 1956.

Bennett, W. A. Students, patients share halfway house. *Rehabilitation Record*, 1964, 5(2), 21–23.

Bettelheim, B. *Love is not enough*. Glencoe, Ill.: Free Press, 1950.

Bettelheim, B. *The informed heart*. Glencoe, Ill.: Free Press, 1960.

Black, B. J. The workaday world: some problems in return of mental patients to the community. In M. Greenblatt, D. J. Levinson, & R. H. Williams (Eds.), *The patient and the mental hospital*. Glencoe, Ill.: Free Press, 1957. Pp. 577–584.

Black, B. J. The protected workshop. In M. Greenblatt & B. Simon (Eds.), *Rehabilitation of the mentally ill*. Washington, D. C.: American Association for the Advancement of Science, 1959. Pp. 199–211.

Black, B. J., Meyer, H. J., & Borgatta, E. F. Altro health and rehabilitation services: case study of a protected workshop. *Journal of Social Issues*, 1960, 16(2) 40–46.

Blacker, E., & Kantor, D. Half-way houses for problem drinkers. *Federal Probation*, 1960, 24(2), 18–23.

Bockoven, J. S. Some relationships between cultural attitudes toward individuality and care of the mentally ill: an historical study. In M. Greenblatt, D. J. Levinson, & R. H. Williams (Eds.), *The patient and the mental hospital*. Glencoe, Ill.: Free Press, 1957. Pp. 517–526.

Bowen, M. A family concept of schizophrenia. In D. D. Jackson (Ed.), *The Etiology of schizophrenia*. New York: Basic Books, 1960. Pp. 346–372.

Breslin, M. A., & Crosswhite, R. G. Residential aftercare: an intermediate step in the correctional process. *Federal Probation*, 1963, **27**(1), 37–46.

Brooks, G. W. Opening a rehabilitation house. In M. Greenblatt, & B. Simon (Eds.) *Rehabilitation of the mentally ill*. Washington, D. C.: American Association for the Advancement of Science, 1959. Pp. 127–139.

Brooks, G. W. Rehabilitation of hospitalized chronic schizophrenia patients. In L. Appleby, J. M. Scher, & J. Cumming, *Chronic schizophrenia*. Glencoe, Ill.: Free Press, 1960. Pp. 248–257.

Brooks, G. W. Rural community influences and supports in a rehabilitation program for state hospital patients. In M. Greenblatt, D. J. Levinson, & G. L. Klerman (Eds.), *Mental patients in transition; steps in hospital-community rehabilitation*. Springfield, Ill.: Charles C Thomas, 1961. Pp. 133–138.

Caplan, G. Mental health consultation in schools. In Milbank Memorial Fund (Ed.), *The elements of a community mental health program*. New York: Milbank Memorial Fund, 1956. Pp. 75–85.

Caudill, W. *The psychiatric hospital as a small society*. Cambridge, Mass.: Harvard University Press, 1958.

Caudill, W., & Stainbrook, E. Some covert effects of communication difficulties in a psychiatric hospital. *Psychiatry*, 1954, **17**, 27–40.

Chittick, R. A., Brooks, G. W., Irons, F. S., & Deane, W. N. The Vermont story: rehabilitation of chronic schizoprhenic patients. Burlington, Vt.: Queen City Printers, 1961.

Conard House, Second Progress Report. Unpublished manuscript, Conard House, San Francisco, February, 1963.

Cumming, J., & Cumming, Elaine. Social equilibrium and social change in the large mental hospital. In M. Greenblatt, D. J. Levinson, & R. H. Williams (Eds.), *The patient and the mental hospital*. Glencoe, Ill.: Free Press, 1957. Pp. 49–72.

Cumming, J., & Cumming, Elaine. *Ego and milieu. Theory and practice of environmental therapy*. New York: Atherton Press, 1962.

Dohan, J. L. Development of a student volunteer program in a state mental hospital. In M. Greenblatt, D. J. Levinson, & R. H. Williams, (Eds.), *The patient and the mental hospital*. Glencoe, Ill.: Free Press, 1957. Pp. 593–603.

Doniger, Joan. Paper presented at the meeting of the New York State Mental Health Association, Buflalo, April 1964.

Doniger, Joan, Rothwell, Naomi, D., & Cohen, R. Case study of a halfway house. *Mental Hospitals*, 1963, **14**, 191–199.

Duhl, L. J. (Ed.) *The urban condition.* New York: Basic Books, 1963.

Eissler, K. R. The effect of the structure of the ego on psychoanalytic technique. *Journal of the American Psychoanalytic Association,* 1953, 1, 104–143.

Erikson, E. H. *Childhood and society.* New York: Norton, 1950.

Erikson, E. H. Identity and the life cycle. *Psychological Issues,* 1959, 1, 1–171.

Erikson, E. H. *Insight and responsibility; lectures on the ethical implications of psychoanalytic insight.* New York: Norton, 1964.

Erikson, K. T., Sharp, G. A. & Maeda, Edith. Profile of a halfway house. Report on Project Grant MH 00454-03, National Institute of Mental Health, 1963.

Fairweather, G. W. (Ed.) *Social psychology in treating mental illness: an experimental approach.* New York: Wiley, 1964.

Farber, L. The therapeutic despair. In L. Farber, *The ways of the will.* New York: Basic Books, 1966. Pp. 155–183. (a)

Farber, L. Schizophrenia and the mad psychotherapist In L. Farber, *The ways of the will.* New York: Basic Books, 1966. Pp. 184–208. (b)

Faris, R. E. L., & Dunham, H. W. *Mental disorders in urban areas.* Chicago: University of Chicago Press, 1939.

Federn, P. *Ego psychology and the psychoses.* New York: Basic Books, 1952.

Fishman, J. R., Pearl, A., & MacLennan, B. New careers—ways out of poverty for disadvantaged youth. Washington, D. C.: Howard University Center for Youth and Community Studies, March 1965.

Flavell, J. H. *The developmental psychology of Jean Piaget.* Princeton, N. J.: Van Nostrand, 1963.

Fountain House Foundation, Inc. Progress Report, 1965. Brochure prepared by Fountain House Foundation, New York, 1965.

Freeman, H. E., & Simmons, O. G. *The mental patient comes home.* New York: Wiley, 1963.

Freud, S. Analysis terminable and interminable (1937). In Freud, S., *Collected papers.* Vol. V. London: Hogarth, 1950. Pp. 316–358.

Freud, S. The interpretation of dreams (1900). In *The complete psychological works of Sigmund Freud.* Vol. V. London: Hogarth, 1953.

Freud, S. *The origins of psychoanalysis. Letters to Wilhelm Fliess, drafts and notes: 1887–1902.* London: Imago Publishing, 1954.

Fromm-Reichmann, Frieda. *Principles of intensive psychotherapy.* Chicago: University of Chicago Press, 1950.

Galioni, E. F., Notman, R. R., Stanton, A. H., & Williams, R. H. The nature and purposes of mental hospital wards. In M. Greenblatt, D. J. Levinson, & R. H. Williams (Eds.), *The patient and the mental hospital*. Glencoe, Ill.: Free Press, 1957. Pp. 327–356.

Ghan, S. L. The "halfway house": a transitional facility for the rehabilitation of the mentally ill—a comparative analytical survey of North American examples. Unpublished master's thesis, University of British Columbia, 1962.

Goertzel, V., Beard, J. H., & Pilnick, S. Fountain House Foundation: case study of an expatient's club. *Journal of Social Issues*, 1960, 16(2), 54–61.

Goffman, E. *Asylums: essays on the social situation of mental patients and other inmates*. Garden City, N. Y.: Doubleday, 1961.

Gomness, C. D. Supervision of Rutland Corner House: a transitional residence. In M. Greenblatt, D. J. Levinson, & G. L. Klerman (Eds.), *Mental patients in transition; steps in hospital-community rehabilitation*. Springfield, Ill.: Charles C Thomas, 1961. Pp. 83–88.

Goodrich, D. W. Possibilities for preventive intervention during initial personality formation. In G. Caplan (Ed.), *Prevention of mental disorders in children*. New York: Basic Books, 1961. Pp. 249–264.

Goodrich, D. W., & Boomer, D. S. Some concepts about therapeutic interventions with hyperaggressive children. Parts I and II. *Social Casework*, 1958, 39, 207–213 and 286–291.

Greenblatt, M. Levinson, D. J., & Klerman, G. L. (Eds.) *Mental patients in transition; steps in hospital-community rehabilitation*. Springfield, Ill.: Charles C Thomas, 1961.

Greenblatt, M., Levinson, D. J., & Williams, R. H. (Eds.) *The patient and the mental hospital*. Glencoe, Ill.: Free Press, 1957.

Greenblatt, M., & Lidz, T. Some dimensions of the problem. In M. Greenblatt, D. J. Levinson, & R. H. Williams (Eds.), *The patient and the mental hospital*. Glencoe, Ill.: Free Press, 1957. Pp. 501–526.

Greenblatt, M., & Simon, B. (Eds.) *Rehabilitation of the mentally ill*. Washington, D. C.: American Association for the Advancement of Science, 1959.

Greenblatt, M., York, R. H., & Brown, Esther L. *From custodial to therapeutic patient care in mental hospitals*. New York: Rusell Sage Foundation, 1955.

Gumrukcu, Patricia, & Mikels, Elaine. Combating post-hospital bends: patterns of success and failure in a psychiatric halfway house. *Mental Hygiene*, 1965, 49, 244–249.

Gurin, G., Veroff, J., & Feld, Sheila. *Americans view their mental health: a nationwide interview survey.* New York: Basic Books, 1960.

Gutman House, Progress Report, February 1963. Demonstration Grant, Office of Vocational Rehabilitation.

Hamburg, D. A. Therapeutic aspects of communication and administrative policy in the psychiatric section of a general hospital. In M. Greenblatt, D. J. Levinson, & R. H. Williams (Eds.), *The patient and the mental hospital.* Glencoe, Ill.: Free Press, 1957. Pp. 91–107.

Henry, G. W. Mental hospitals. In G. Zilboorg, *A history of medical psychology.* New York: Norton, 1941. Pp. 558–589.

Henry, J. The formal structure of a psychiatric hospital. *Psychiatry,* 1954, **17**, 139–152.

Henry, J. Types of institutional structure. In M. Greenblatt, D. J. Levinson, & R. H. Williams (Eds.), *The patient and the mental hospital.* Glencoe, Ill.: Free Press, 1957. Pp. 73–90.

Heron, W. The pathology of boredom. *Scientific American,* 1957, **196**, 52–56.

Hollingshead, A. G., & Redlich, F. C. *Social class and mental illness. A community study.* New York: Wiley, 1958.

Huseth, B. England's halfway houses. *Mental Hospitals,* 1962, **13**, 422–424.

Jackson, D. D. (Ed.) *The etiology of schizophrenia.* New York: Basic Books, 1960.

Jones, E. *The life and work of Sigmund Freud.* New York: Basic Books, 1953.

Jones, M. *The therapeutic community.* New York: Basic Books, 1953.

Journal of Social Issues. New pathways from the mental hospital. *Journal of Social Issues,* 1960, **16**(2), 1–80.

Kantor, D., & Gelineau, V. Wellmet, halfway house for chronic mental patients—a Harvard-Radcliffe student volunteer program, Progress Report, March 1963. Demonstration Grant, Office of Vocational Rehabilitation.

Kantor, D., & Greenblatt, M. Wellmet: halfway to community rehaiblitation. *Mental Hospitals,* 1962, **13**, 146–151.

Kennard, E. A. Psychiatry, administrative psychiatry, administration: a study of a veterans hospital. In M. Greenblatt, D. J. Levinson, & R. H. Williams (Eds.), *The patient and the mental hospital.* Glencoe, Ill.: Free Press, 1957. Pp. 36–45.

Kesey, K. *One flew over the cuckoo's nest.* New York: Viking Press, 1962.

Klerman, G. L. Historical baselines for the evaluation of maintenance drug therapy of discharged psychiatric patients. In M. Greenblatt, D. J. Levinson, & G. L. Klerman (Eds.), *Mental patients in transition; steps in hospital-community rehabilitation.* Springfield, Ill.: Charles C Thomas, 1961. Pp. 287–301.

Kling, V. G. Space: a fundamental concept in design. In C. E. Goshen, *Psychiatric architecture.* Washington, D. C.: American Psychiatric Association, 1959.

Knight, R. P. Psychotherapy of an adolescent catatonic schizophrenic with mutism; a study in empathy and establishing contact. *Psychiatry,* 1946, 9, 323–339.

Kohler, L. H., Bandle, D. F., Ossorio, A. G., & Schumacher, B. Rehabilitation house for psychiatric patients. St. Louis State Hospital Progress Report, February 1962. Research and Demonstration Grant 630, Office of Vocational Rehabilitation.

Kohn, M. L. Social class and parental values. *American Journal of Sociology,* 1959, 64, 337–351.

Landy, D. Rutland Corner House: case study of a halfway house. *Journal of Social Issues,* 1960, 16(2), 27–32.

Landy, D. A halfway house for women: preliminary report of a study. In M. Greenblatt, D. J. Levinson, & G. L. Klerman (Eds.), *Mental patients in transition; steps in hospital-community rehabilitation.* Springfield, Ill.: Charles C Thomas, 1961. Pp. 94–103.

Landy, D., & Greenblatt, M. *Halfway house.* A sociocultural and clinical study of Rutland Corner House, a transitional aftercare residence for female psychiatric patients. United States Department of Health, Education, and Welfare; Vocational Rehabilitation Administration, 1965.

Landy, D., & Raulet, H. The hospital work program. In M. Greenblatt, & B. Simon (Eds.), *Rehabilitation of the mentally ill.* Washington, D. C.: American Association for the Advancement of Science, 1959. Pp. 71–87.

Lidz, T., Fleck, S., Cornelison, Alice R., with the collaboration of Alanen, Y. O., and others. *Schizophrenia and the family.* New York: International Universities Press, 1965.

Lindemann, E. Symptomatology and management of acute grief. *American Journal of Psychiatry,* 1944, 101, 141–148.

Lindemann, E. Psycho-social factors as stressor agents. In J. M. Tanner (Ed.), *Stress and psychiatric disorder.* Oxford: Blackwell Scientific Publications, 1960.

Lurie, A., & Pinsky, Louise. Collaboration between psychiatric hospital and community agencies in the rehabilitation of mental patients. In M. Greenblatt, D. J. Levinson, & G. L. Klerman (Eds.), *Mental patients in transition; steps in hospital-community rehabilitation.* Springfield, Ill.: Charles C Thomas, 1961. Pp. 163–174.

Lyman, Susan. History and organization of the Rutland Corner (halfway) House. In M. Greenblatt, D. J. Levinson, & G. L. Klerman (Eds.), *Mental patients in transition; steps in hospital-community rehabilitation.* Springfield, Ill.: Charles C Thomas, 1961. Pp. 77–82.

Maeda, Edith M., & Rothwell, Naomi D. Discussion, listing and bibliography of psychiatric halfway houses in the United States. Psychiatric Studies and Projects, No. 9. Washington, D. C.: Mental Hospital Service of the American Psychiatric Association, September, 1963.

Meenach, L. The stepping stone. A report of residential rehabilitation houses for the mentally ill. March 1964, VRA Grant RD-566-60. Frankfort, Kentucky: State Department of Education, Bureau of Rehabilitation Services.

Menninger, K. Concerning our advocacy of a unitary concept of mental illness. In L. Appleby, J. M. Scher, & J. Cumming, *Chronic schizophrenia.* Glencoe, Ill.: Free Press, 1960. Pp. 54–67.

Menninger, K., Ellenberger, H., Pruyser, P., & Mayman, M. The unitary concept of mental illness. *Bulletin of the Menninger Foundation,* 1958, **22,** 4–12.

Mikels, Elaine, & Gumrukcu, Patricia. A therapeutic halfway hostel. *Mental Hospitals,* 1963, **14,** 219. (a)

Mikels, Elaine, & Gumrukcu, Patricia. Conard House—bridge to reality. *Rehabilitation Record,* 1963, **4**(4), 24–27. (b)

Miller, D. R., & Swanson, G. E. *The changing American parent.* New York: Wiley, 1958.

Neff, W. S. Research needs and perspectives. *Rehabilitation Record,* 1964, **5**(2), 17–20.

Olshansky, S. Employer receptivity. In M. Greenblatt, & B. Simon (Eds.), *Rehabilitation of the mentally ill.* Washington, D. C. American Association for the Advancement of Science, 1959. Pp. 213–221.

Olshansky, S. The transitional sheltered workshop: a survey. *Journal of Social Issues,* 1960, **16**(2), 33–39.

Parsons, T. The mental hospital as a type of organization. In M. Greenblatt, D. J. Levinson, & R. H. Williams (Eds.), *The patient and the mental hospital.* Glencoe, Ill.: Free Press, 1957. Pp. 108–129.

Pinel, P. See G. Zilboorg, *A history of medical psychology*. New York: Norton, 1941. Pp. 319–341.

Polansky, N. A., White, R. B., & Miller, S. C. Determinants of the role-image of the patient in a psychiatric hospital. In M. Greenblatt, D. J. Levinson, & R. H. Williams (Eds.), *The patient and the mental hospital*. Glencoe, Ill.: Free Press, 1957. Pp. 380–401.

Rapaport, R. N. *Community as doctor. New perspectives on a therapeutic community*. Springfield, Ill.: Charles C Thomas, 1960.

Redl, F. Strategies and techniques of the life-space interview. *American Journal of Orthopsychiatry*, 1959, **29**, 1–18. (a)

Redl, F. The concept of a "therapeutic milieu". *American Journal of Orthopsychiatry*, 1959, **29**, 721–736. (b)

Redl, F. *When we deal with children: selected writings*. New York: Free Press, 1966.

Redl, F., & Wineman, D. *Children who hate*. Glencoe, Ill.: Free Press, 1951.

Redl, F., & Wineman, D. *Controls from within: techniques for the treatment of the aggressive child*. Glencoe, Ill.: Free Press, 1952.

Reiff, R. Mental health manpower and institutional change. *American Psychologist*, 1966, **21**, 540–548.

Reik, L. E. The halfway house: the role of laymen's organizations in the rehabilitation of the mentally ill. *Mental Hygiene*, 1953, **37**, 615–618.

Robinson, R., deMarche, D. F., & Wagle, M. K. *Community resources in mental health*. Joint Commission on Mental Illness and Health, Monograph Series No. 5. New York: Basic Books, 1960.

Rosen, J. N. *Direct analysis: selected papers*. New York: Grune & Stratton, 1953.

Rosenthal, D. (Ed.) *The Genain quadruplets*. New York: Basic Books, 1963.

Rothwell, Naomi D., & Doniger, Joan. Halfway house and mental hospital—some comparisons. *Psychiatry*, 1963, **26**, 281–288.

Rothwell, Naomi D., & Doniger, Joan M. *The psychiatric halfway house. A case study*. Springfield, Ill.: Charles C Thomas, 1966.

Schwartz, M. S., & Schwartz, Charlotte G. *Social aproaches to mental patient care*. New York: Columbia University Press, 1964.

Sechehaye, Marguerite A. *Symbolic realization*. New York: International Universities Press, 1951.

Shaw, Judith. Follow-up after the halfway house. *Rehabilitation Record*, 1965, **6**(2), 29–30.

Sivadon, P. D. Techniques of sociotherapy. *Psychiatry*, 1957, **20**, 205–210.

Smith, Dorothy E. The logic of custodial organization. *Psychiatry*, 1965, **28**, 311–324.

Smith, M. B., & Hobbs, N. The community and the community mental health center. *American Psychologist*, 1966, **21**, 499–509.

Stanton, A. H., & Schwartz, M. S. *The mental hospital.* Glencoe, Ill.: Basic Books, 1954.

Sullivan, H. S. *The interpersonal theory of psychiatry.* New York: Norton, 1953.

Szasz, T. *The myth of mental illness: foundations of a theory of personal conduct.* New York: Harper & Row, 1961.

Thibaut, J. W., & Kelley, H. H. *The social psychology of groups.* New York: Wiley, 1959.

Thomas, E. J., & Fink, C. F. Effects of group size. *Psychological Bulletin*, 1963, **60**, 371–384.

Umbarger, C. C. Prepared with the assistance of D. Kantor and M. Greenblatt. *College students in a mental hospital.* New York: Grune & Stratton, 1962.

van den Berg, J. H. *The changing nature of man.* New York: Norton, 1961.

von Mering, O., & King, S. H. *Remotivating the mental patient.* New York: Russell Sage Foundation, 1957.

Washburn, S. L., & DeVore, I. The social life of baboons. *Scientific American*, 1961, **204**(6), 62–71.

Wayne, G. J. The special contributions of a hospital halfway house. *Mental Hospitals*, 1963, **14**, 440–442.

Wechsler, H. Halfway houses for former mental patients: a survey. *Journal of Social Issues*, 1960, **16**(2), 20–26.

Wellmet, halfway house for chronic mental patients—a Harvard-Radcliffe student volunteer program. Progress Report, March 1963. Demonstration Grant, Office of Vocational Rehabilitation.

Werner, H. *Comparative psychology of mental development.* New York: International Universities Press, 1957.

Will, O. A. Process, psychotherapy, and schizophrenia. In A. Burton (Ed.), *Psychotherapy of the psychoses.* New York: Basic Books, 1961. Pp. 10–42.

Wilmer, H. A. Graphic ways of representing some aspects of a therapeutic community. In *Symposium on preventive and social psychiatry*, sponsored jointly by the Walter Reed Army Institute of Research, Walter Reed Army Medical Center, and the National Research Council, Washington, D. C., April 1957. Pp. 465–478.

Wilmer, H. A. *Social psychiatry in action: a therapeutic community.* Springfield, Ill.: Charles C Thomas, 1958.

Woodley House, Annual Report. Unpublished manuscript. Woodley House, Washington, D. C., 1965.

Woodley House Conference on Halfway Houses, Charlotte L. Raush. Held in May 1963. Unpublished manuscript, Woodley House, Washington, D. C.

Wynne, L., Ryckoff, I., Day, Juliana, & Hirsch, S. Pseudo-mutuality in the family relations of schizophrenics. *Psychiatry,* 1958, **21**, 205–220.

Wynne, L., & Singer, Margaret. Thought disorders and the family relations of schizophrenics: I. A research strategy. *Archives of General Psychiatry,* 1963, 9, 191–198. (a)

Wynne, L., & Singer, Margaret. Thought disorders and family relations of schizophrenics: II. A classification of forms of thinking. *Archives of General Psychiatry,* 1963, 9, 199–206. (b)

Zilboorg, G. *A history of medical psychology.* New York: Norton, 1941.

INDEX OF AUTHORS

INDEX OF SUBJECTS